OLDER AND WIDER

A Survivor's Guide to the Menopause

Jenny Eclair

Quercus

Hardback edition published in Great Britain in 2020 by Quercus Editions Ltd

This paperback edition published in 2021 by

Quercus Editions Ltd
Carmelite House
50 Victoria Embankment
London EC4Y oDZ

An Hachette UK company

A CIP catalogue record for this book is available
from the British Library

PB ISBN 978 1 52940 357 2
Ebook ISBN 978 1 52940 356 5

Every effort has been made to contact copyright holders.
However, the publishers will be glad to rectify in future editions
any inadvertent omissions brought to their attention.

Quercus Editions Ltd hereby exclude all liability to the extent permitted by law
for any errors or omissions in this book and for any loss, damage or expense
(whether direct or indirect) suffered by a third party relying on
any information contained in this book.

If you have a medical condition or suspect one, consult your GP.
Nothing in this book is intended to replace or override any medical advice or
treatment you may be receiving. Author and publisher accept no responsibility
for health outcomes from the information contained in this book.

10 9 8 7 6 5 4 3 2 1

Typeset by CC Book Production
Printed and bound in Great Britain by Clays Ltd, Elcograf S.p.A.

MIX
Paper from
responsible sources
FSC® C104740

Papers used by Quercus are from well-managed forests and other responsible sources.

This book is dedicated to all the menopausal women out there.

Because there are loads of us scurrying around in a furious temper, faces like hammerhead sharks, wondering what the hell to have for tea. All with a combined temperature of a billion trillion degrees.

HOW IT ALL STARTS

'Ladies, just remember, you're not alone. There's millions of us and we're all in this leaky old boat together.' JE

Hello, welcome to *Older and Wider* – every menopausal woman's A–Z compendium of the menopause.

If you're after an in-depth medical/psychological insight into the menopause, I'm afraid you've opened the wrong book – I'm not a doctor . . . Oh, hold on, I am. I got one of those mad honorary degrees from Middlesex University! So officially, I'm Dr Jenny Eclair, but unfortunately, they didn't give me a prescription pad or a stethoscope, and let's just say that if anyone ever shouts for a doctor in an emergency, it's best I don't step forward.

However, I am a woman and I do know how it feels to be menopausal, so this book is written from experience and the heart and I hope it makes you laugh and feel better. Laughing at anything that upsets, rattles and derails us is one of the first steps towards dealing with it, being able to put it into context. A problem shared and all that, which is why it's important that we are able to talk about it without fear of upsetting or embarrassing anyone. Personally, I can't see what's embarrassing about the female ageing process anyway. It's not as if blokes age with any more dignity than we do; let's face it, most of them have turned into human Toby jugs by the time they've hit sixty.

One of the simple facts of life is that more or less half the world's population will go through the menopause and yet, apparently, in some circles the subject is still considered taboo. Now I don't mix in those circles, because I live in the twenty-first century and not in 1957. I belong to a world of stroppy, hard-working women who don't really have the time or the inclination to play the shy, retiring violet.

Us ladies have changed. We no longer wear hats and girdles – we're letting it all hang out –and we're no longer whispering behind closed doors about our 'down theres'.

Of course, there are some people who would rather turn the clock back, and I imagine that somewhere in the dusty back rooms of certain types of gentlemen's clubs there are still a handful of florid-faced men who still gag at the mention of anything so intimately female and middle-aged. 'The menopause?' (Harrumph, shuffle *Daily Telegraph*, sip single malt.) 'Why do the ladies have to make such a song and dance about it? Why are their bodies so complicated and messy? And why don't they put up the toilet seat after they've finished doing whatever disgusting thing they've been doing in there?'

Like something from *The Fast Show*, these are the type of dinosaur men who reckon women should put up and shut up, just like they did in the olden days, biting down on wooden spoons and taking secret swigs of cooking sherry when things got tough.

Well, sorry, chaps. The fairer sex are no longer content to boil silently and uncomplainingly in the corner. We're having a hard time over here and the least you can do is man up and open that tricky sash window for us. And no, you don't need to worry; we're not going to jump out of it – we just want some fresh air and a little bit of understanding.

As long as there has been life on earth, then, there have been menopausal women, stomping about, feeling furious, giving the old man grief for bringing home some scraggy bit of flea-bitten mammoth and complaining about 'the bloody fire being too hot'.

The most unusual thing about the menopause is how few animals experience it. Most species are designed to breed until they die! Thank heavens for small mercies, eh, because the idea of dropping sprogs in my eighties fills me with horror (seriously, I'd really rather be watching *Countdown* than changing nappies).

Apart from us, the only other mammals who lose the ability to breed and yet continue to live, are the short-finned pilot whale and her bigger sister, the killer whale.

Speaking for myself, I find the idea of a menopausal killer whale incredibly appealing. I like picturing the whopping thing having a massive strop in the middle of the ocean, steam rising from her blowholes, all the other fish keeping well clear, plankton swimming for their lives.

A possible theory behind the killer whale's menopause is that the older, non-breeding matriarch, once free from looking after babies, is available to keep an eye on her older offspring who are apt to perish without Mum being there to show them where the salmon is.

Typical, isn't it? Looks like it's not just our reproductive habits that we share with the lady whales; on top of everything else, us middle-aged women are the only ones with that killer supermarket instinct – without us, the rest of the family would, no doubt, starve to death.

Once upon a time, people could plead menopause ignorance. In the 1970s, very few men had heard of the word oestrogen and those who had thought it was an Austrian lager. Whilst it was fine for TV commercials to feature young women hand-rolling cigars suggestively on their inner thighs, anything to do with the ageing female reproductive system was kept strictly under wraps. In fact, during my 'health and hygiene' classes at school, there was some sketchy information about periods, intercourse, STIs and pregnancy, but the menopause was never mentioned. Which was a shame, considering that half the teachers at Queen Mary's girls' grammar were obviously in the grip of some kind of hormonal turmoil and we might have had a tad more sympathy for them if we'd known what they were going through. No wonder one of the teachers kept a quart of vodka tucked away inside the baby grand.

The menopause can be quite a tricky subject to pin down. There are no rights and wrongs, and certainly no rules. No two women will have identical symptoms – in that respect the menopause is a bit of a moveable feast – and the message I'm trying to get across in this book is that there's no such thing as normal.

How we deal with this chunk of our lives isn't helped if you feel that no one else is going through what you are going through. And this is the biggest menopausal myth that needs busting. As I write this, there are currently 13 million women in the UK who are menopausal or peri-menopausal – that's a hell of a big gang to belong to and we all need to take comfort from this fact and keep sharing our problems and experiences.

These days, although people are much more relaxed about the subject, the menopause genie still seems slightly wedged in the neck of her bottle: she's not completely 'out'. But thanks to the Internet and a new wave of TV programmes and speciality podcasts, progress is being made. Women are even allowed to speak of dry vaginas on pre-watershed telly (more on this later) and no amount of shuffling newspapers and harrumphing is going to drown us out.

And the really great thing about the menopause today is that, rather than die of shame for daring to mention the M word out loud, we're allowed to make jokes about it. Personally, I think the more jokes the better; there's nothing more off-putting than a slightly hushed mealy-mouthed and earnest approach to the subject. What we don't need are more statistics and dry medical data that are going to scare the shit out of everyone. We want a bit of light and humanity shining on all this. And hopefully a few laughs – because there are silver linings, I promise.

The conversation has begun, and as long as women continue to wake up feeling weepy in a sweat-soaked nightie at 3am, it's in everyone's best interests to listen.

A

ARE YOU SURE YOU'RE MENOPAUSAL?

'Denial is a wonderful thing, but at some point you will have to accept that it isn't normal to be stripping off your cardigan when everybody else is huddling around the radiator.' **JE**

First of all, are you sure you're menopausal? Here's a quick tick list:

- Do you have tampons gathering dust at the bottom of your handbag?
- Has your hormone-tracking app gone into meltdown?
- Do people think you've just got out of the shower because 'you look a bit hot'?

Congratulations and welcome to the club!

There's a great deal of stereotyping when it comes to the image of the menopausal woman. But the fact is, whilst many of us tick at least some of the usual boxes – hot, frazzled, fat and bad-tempered – others (slightly annoyingly for the rest of us) reach menopausal age still looking like they could easily slip into their old school uniforms and sneak undetected into a local sixth-form common room.

Darcey Bussell and Tess Daly both turned fifty in 2019! I know, right? Give the rest of us a break, girls. Tess was pictured recently on her hols in a bikini top and wearing a teeny tiny pair of pink shorts, whilst Darcey still has the legs of a gazelle. Neither of them fits the conventional image of the miserable middle-aged old bag who has just left a packet of mince at the checkout and is having a meltdown on the 176 bus (guilty). But it just goes to show that women are all different, and all will approach the menopause in their own sweet way. One size does not fit all, as anyone who has ever attempted to try on Tess Daly's shorts will tell you.

WHAT'S YOUR TYPE?

How you deal with the arrival of your menopause will depend on many things: whether you've been expecting it, if it's medically induced, the severity of your symptoms (it's an undeniable truth that some women suffer more than others) and the type of person you are.

The world of women divides into those who naturally cope and those who flap and panic. On a sliding scale of coping, with stoicism at one end and full-blown hysteria at the other, I am probably somewhere around the middle. But let's face it, even those born with a stiff upper lip have to let it wobble now and then; after all, the menopause isn't like having a three-day cold – you can't retire under the duvet with a really good box set and wait for the worst to be over. Not unless you fancy spending up to a decade in bed. Hmmmmmmm?

So how will *you* cope? Well, that depends on which one of the following best sums you up.

THE GIRL GUIDE

We all know a girl-guide type. She's the one who has a cagoule for every occasion and an emergency piece of Kendal Mint Cake in her pocket at all times. She is capable and practical and knows which direction the sun will rise in and whether your garden is south-facing. These are the women for whom the motto 'Be prepared' might as well be tattooed across their foreheads.

The girl guide goes through life cheerfully facing challenges head on. She actually likes sleeping under canvas, knows all the words to 'She'll be coming round the mountain' and doesn't automatically want to kill people who bring out acoustic guitars at social gatherings. She can catch a fish with a safety pin and a suspender belt and, what's more, she can gut it and fry it for breakfast, on a fire she has lit herself, sans matches, by rubbing two sticks together and igniting a bit of old sheep's wool and some kindling. The girl guide is the least squeamish of all your mates. She is the one who has done the first-aid course and has the badge to prove it; she came into her own that time at Sue's fiftieth birthday party when Janet started choking on a bit of sausage roll and she performed the Heimlich manoeuvre on her on the dance floor and everyone cheered when a piece of puff pastry shot out of Janet's gullet and she lived to do the Macarena one more time.

Goddammit . . . The menopause isn't going to beat the girl guide. She's read the books, she knows the drill, she's already bought a lightweight summer duvet from Peter Jones in case she starts over-heating in the night, she's made sure all the upstairs sash windows are fully operational and has practised sleeping in the altogether, in the draught between the bedroom and the bathroom. For her, preparing for the menopause will be a reminder of the giddy excitement of training for her Duke of Edinburgh award; it's just another challenge along life's long yomp.

Our girl guide will have processed all relevant data and popped a memo in her diary to expect the arrival of the menopause somewhere around her fifty-first birthday. To be on the safe side, she's upped her supplement intake (multivitamins and iron) and tweaked her diet to deal with any encroaching hormonal onslaught. She has even phoned her mother (AKA the Guide captain) to ask her when *she* stopped menstruating (a tricky conversation, considering neither has spoken about anything below the panty line before in their lives, but needs must).

After all, 'forewarned is forearmed' and, of course, the most important thing is not to panic. What's the worst the menopause can do? It can't be worse than stepping into a really deep bog and spending the rest of the day with wet socks, or bungee jumping off the O2 or wing-walking on a World War II spitfire (both of which she's done for charity without breaking sweat).

Of course, when the menopause does hit, the girl guide will be the one who unexpectedly finds herself on her knees having a crisis of confidence and crying over whether to put blueberries or banana on her breakfast porridge. The physical effects of the much-anticipated hot flush won't be a problem, but what will really throw her is the fact that, without warning, her brain will seem foggier than that time she got lost on top of Ben Nevis in a freezing pea souper with nothing but a compass she got out of a crappy Christmas cracker for guidance. Suddenly, every decision – be it what to have for supper, where to go on holiday or even which top to wear today – will seem insurmountable. For someone who has always been pretty snappy when it comes to making choices, this will be uncharted territory. (If you've never been a ditherer before and then you find yourself stuck in Sainsbury's with a cauliflower in one hand and a cabbage in the other, frozen with indecision, then this will be your cue to take a hike down to see your local GP.)

THE MENOPAUSAL CELEBRITY

In the old days, celebrities didn't have the menopause. For years, the only actresses ever to appear on screen in rabidly hormonal mode were Bette Davis and Joan Crawford in *What Ever Happened to Baby Jane?* Even now, in these more enlightened times there are still a few celebs for whom admitting they are exactly the same as everyone else is a no-no.

For starters, our menopausal celebrity won't expect it to happen to her, not until she's well into her sixties. After all, she can still get away with long hair and wearing white jeans, plus she's got a swim-wear collection to flog.

Of course, things will take a tricky turn when the old periods start arriving out of the blue and all of a sudden wearing white jeans and skimpy swimwear are off the agenda, given she needs several heavy-duty Dr Whites anchored permanently into her knickers. In fact, for the first time in her life the menopausal celebrity will have to buy a proper pair of knickers complete with a backside to which she can adhere said sanitary towels rather than the non-protective, buttock-exposing thong of old. Still, this will be the menopausal celebrity's first perk of the process – for the first time in thirty-five years she is wearing comfy pants.

Of course, her biggest problem – apart from suddenly getting very sweaty, which she puts down to just having 'jogged here', despite wearing Louboutin six-inch heels – is whether to keep schtum. Should she visit that Botox bloke off Harley Street (the one everyone else goes to but pretends they don't) and deny all knowledge of any change in the downstairs area, or should she come out as a brave menopausal pioneer and hopefully get a round of chat shows out of it?

In the end, she will probably have to come clean after one of those hideous celebrity magazines takes a photo of her looking a bit haggard and buying a packet of TENA Lady in the supermarket. At this point, the offers for discreet lady products will come flooding in and she will not know whether to laugh or cry (which, of course, is another common menopause symptom). But instead of nipping down to her NHS doctor's surgery for a bit of a chat, our menopausal celebrity will find the 'best' gynae expert in town (usually via the back pages of *Tatler*) and will end up having a consultation in a smart room with fresh orchids on the desk, free coffee and a selection of magazines, none of which will be more than a month out of date. Our celebrity will be on first-name terms with her gynaecologist, they will air kiss each other and she will be prescribed a course of bioidentical hormones, rather than the bog-standard HRT the rest of us get (according to folklore, pregnant horse urine is said to be involved in the cheap stuff).

Our menopausal sleb will be utterly thrilled with her medication; her skin will glow, her hair will be lusher than ever and normal oh-so-sexy service will be resumed. However, the one big lifestyle change she will make will concern her pants – she will never return to thongs again; from now on she will be a big-panted woman.

NOTTING HILL PERI-MENOPAUSAL PRINCESS

It might come as a surprise to many, but even thin, rich women who live in those massive white houses in Notting Hill – the ones that look like wedding cakes – go through the change too. They just do it in more expensive yoga pants.

Our Notting Hill peri-menopausal princess who juices, meditates and very occasionally eats lunch will find the whole process rather trying and traumatic because it's one of the very few things in her life that she actually has to do herself. Everything else that's boring and hard work she pays a minion to do. Ironing, cleaning, looking after the children – all those tedious little jobs she doesn't fancy – are done by a team of other women. Sadly, it is impossible to pay another woman to go through the menopause for you. No matter how much money you have in the world, you cannot have a menopause surrogate.

Once she gets over the horror of not being able to employ a girl to do it for her, our Notting Hill peri-menopausal princess will start taking her menopause very seriously indeed. In fact, sod Buddhism, the menopause, peri and beyond, will become her new religion. She might even have her interiors repainted by someone who specializes in 'hormone harmony for the house'. Whilst indoors is being painted in gentle tones of vulval pink, our princess will spend a couple of weeks alongside other like-minded thin, rich women at a menopause retreat in Bali. Here, she will top up her tan and have her oestrogen charts read by a menopause guru. There will also be a great deal of candle-lit chanting, some weeping and hugging and some great cocktails. Once home, there will be a great deal of crystal healing, green-juice drinking and soy substitutes. In fact, a special menopause chef will be installed in the kitchen (although on rare visits to see her children, our Notting Hill peri-menopausal princess will be unable to resist any leftover soggy tomato-sauce-soaked fish fingers and occasionally she will pull up the hood of her Chloe silk parka and sneak off for a bucket of fried chicken which she will eat round the back of some garages). Once the menopause proper kicks in, she will decide to retire from public life, flog the fanny-pink house and move to the country, where she will join the WI and instantly feel ten years younger by simply hanging out with women who *are* ten years older and couldn't give a shit. Within six months, she will have put on two stone, bought a black Labrador, learned to knit and forgotten that she occasionally feels a bit shit.

JO-NORMAL

Having fought a losing battle with the top button of her jeans for weeks, Jo Normal will find herself browsing in Marks looking at nice pull-on trousers and baggy cotton tunic tops. Suddenly, the mere sight of a rail of roll-neck chunky jumpers will bring her out in a massive sweat and she'll be muttering about how 'stupidly hot it is in this place' when she accidentally catches sight of what looks suspiciously like her mum standing just three feet away. Only her mum lives two hundred miles up the M6. Once she realizes that she is, in fact, staring at her own reflection and that she has turned into the doppelganger of her mother in her furious fifties, the truth of what is happening will hit her. Of course, this is it. This is what all those leaflets bang on about. This is what they talk about on *Woman's Hour*. This is the big M.

She is hot, she is chubby, she is bad tempered; the kids are getting on her wick more than normal and she dreads taking her nightie off in the middle of the night in case her old man thinks she's giving him the come on.

At this point, like any sensible fifty-something who realizes the change is upon her, our Jo Normal will march down to the food hall, look for the special offers and buy some nice luxury sausages for tea. Because, let's face it, if you're setting sail into the eye of a hormonal hurricane, then you're going to need some decent sustenance.

Understanding what's wrong can be a big relief for Jo Normal. It means she can go home and tell the family she probably doesn't have a massive brain tumour that is making her behave erratically – she is merely going through what millions of women go through and it means that now and again, they're just going to have to pull their fingers out, help a bit more around the house and put up with the odd rant. Oh yes, and she will occasionally have to open the back door to let in some fresh air and close the bathroom door for a bit of bath time P and Q with a scented candle. Once Jo Normal knows what's going on, she will phone a few mates to see how they're dealing with it, do a quick Google search (without disappearing down a scaremongering wormhole) and make an appointment with her trusty GP to see whether she should go through this cold turkey or what the other options are.

She will also phone her mother and apologize for being a difficult teenage cow whilst her mum went through the menopause all those years ago and then she will put the sausages on, pour a small glass of wine and give herself a private toast.

We all need to put the menopause into perspective. Many of us have lost friends who didn't live long enough to experience it, and whilst the menopause can be gruelling, pegging out before it kicks in is much worse. So next time we're raging on about saggy tits and a lost libido, let's just remember the women who didn't make it to this stage. Then let's all take a deep breath and get on with it.

B

BROODINESS

'One of the tricky aspects of the menopause is how finite it feels. If you imagine your life as a book, then Part One is over and from now on this is Part Two.' **JE**

Of course, there's no reason why Part Two shouldn't be brilliant. But there is also the underlying feeling that this is the bit when you start hurtling towards the end – the menopause is a massive bookmark in your life and sometimes it's hard not to feel broody for your past. Because broodiness isn't all about wanting babies; it's not just about catching sight of a newborn and feeling that tingle in your nipples and a liquid rush of longing in your loins. In truth, I don't get broody over babies any more. These days, if I'm honest, I'd rather have a really great pair of boots.

Broodiness during the menopause can also be a sense of yearning for the life you might have lived, for the chances you let slip through your fingers, the opportunities never grasped and the things you didn't allow yourself to appreciate at the time.

Looking back, with the benefit of age, I realize now that as a younger woman, I rarely celebrated any of my career achievements because as soon as I'd pulled off one trick, I felt everyone expected me to immediately pull off another, each one more impressive than the last.

Older and Wider

I wish now I'd congratulated myself more, but I never dared in case I jinxed myself. It's only as you get older that you realize that your past successes weren't purely down to luck – that they were also down to hard work and tenacity. Sometimes I feel sorry for the young me: I didn't have much cellulite, but I didn't have much confidence either.

When I was thirty-five and had been working as a fully fledged comic for over ten years (previously I'd been a punk poet), I went up to the Edinburgh Festival for the umpteenth time and became the first solo female performer to win a prestigious prize which, at the time, was called the Perrier Award for Best Comedy at the Fringe.

I was blonde, I was attractive, but I was also drinking pretty heavily and the press photos show me looking stunning but a bit mad.

The truth was, I felt mad. I did not feel worthy of the award, yet the night I won it was one of the best of my life. It was everything I'd gone into show business for – popping flashbulbs, bottles of champagne and bouquets of flowers.

But the morning after I felt like hell. I was hungover and paranoid and I only had partial recall of the previous night's celebrations. I knew I'd ended up at a notorious late-night venue (the original Gilded Balloon before it burned down) where I ended up singing onstage with Leo Sayer. Then, because the stilettoes I'd bought for the awards party had made my feet bleed, I'd hitched a ride home to my rented flat, which, in the cold light of day, was full of empty bottles and overflowing ashtrays. All I wanted to do was hide under the duvet. My partner and daughter were hundreds of miles away in Wales, staying at my sister's holiday place, and suddenly I had all these press requests, photo calls and a gig to smash that night. It was ghastly. I wobbled through the last few days of the festival, sobbing on sympathetic strangers' shoulders, babbling rubbish to journalists, sabotaging my own performances and generally hating every minute of being in my own terrified skin.

If I could go back, I'd accept that award and give myself a three-drink limit; then I'd put me in a taxi, take me back to the rented flat, run me a bath, feed me some toast and put me to bed. Maybe then I could have enjoyed my success. Maybe then I would have felt like I deserved it and allowed myself at least a few days of triumph.

Self-preservation is something that took me many years to learn and even now I still don't quite have the hang of it . . . Maybe when I'm older!

WHAT IF?/WHAT NEXT?

Lots of us look back at old photos and wonder why we didn't value what we had at the time.

The trouble with being young is that we never realize quite how gorgeous we are – we're too busy obsessing about how even more gorgeous other people are and taking a magnifying glass to whatever faults we have.

I have a picture on my desk taken in the late 1990s. In it, I'm probably thirty-seven, my partner (who has always been twelve years older) is a well-preserved forty-nine and our daughter is eight. At the time I was doing a great deal of swimming and ashtanga yoga and, boy, does it show. Twenty-plus years later, the old man's hair has gone completely white, I've ballooned and Phoebe has gone from mouse to peroxide blonde.

Older and Wider

Sometimes it's hard to let go of that period in your life when everything is still possible, when it's not too late to have another child or land that career-changing job, when all your options are open, and time and biology are still on your side. There is something very finite about reaching your fifties. Subconsciously, you start imagining that doors are closing. And they are – because let's get real, unless you're going to employ a surrogate, it's highly unlikely you are going to have another child.

When I was in my twenties, I imagined that I would have five children – all little girls with names beginning with P. Optimistically, I hoped they'd be able to sing close harmony and I'd make a fortune out of them. The Eclairettes, I'd call them. As it happened, I managed just the one P-named daughter and despite the fact that I love her more than anything else, I knew by the time I was thirty that Prudence, Pandora, Persephone and Perdita weren't going to happen. I'm still happy with this choice, though I'm not sure she will be when I'm old and gaga.

The other scenario I imagined was that we'd all live in a white stuccoed five-storey Georgian house in Chelsea. Occasionally, even now, I'll be in the neighbourhood and still get this fleeting feeling of what might have been and, for a moment, I can't understand why I don't have the key to one of those big front doors in my handbag.

By the time we are middle-aged, we have turned so many corners it's hard to go back and begin again. We have shaped our futures with the decisions we have made. But that's not to say there aren't exciting things to come, and I refuse to give up on the hope that there are plenty more career opportunities out there.

Nothing sums up the stages in our life like the traditional Russian babushka doll – remember the funny little wooden stacking women that sat on every spoiled girl's windowsill back in the 1970s. I never had one, but even now, given the opportunity I will take one to pieces. We are all our very own babushka dolls: there we are, all neatly stacked inside ourselves, all the versions of us, all intrinsically the same, just tweaked by experience and circumstance, hair dye and fashion. We don't lose the people we used to be; we just swallow them up – they're still inside us.

So yes, whilst occasionally I will find in my wardrobe a little black Muji dress from back in the 1990s that I can no longer get over my arm, I don't want to go back to that time and place. I don't want to be that woman again. She is in me and she's part of me and it's nice to remember the good bits, but considering you can't turn the clock back, there's no point really trying. And anyway, just imagine how thrilled someone will be to find that black size ten Muji number in a charity shop in SE5.

The menopause is a definite chapter in your life. Not only does it mark the end of the young you, it also heralds in the dawn of a new you and what this new you is going to be is very much your decision to make. You've basically got two options: you can be a miserable old cow, furiously looking over your shoulder all the time or you can be one of those infuriatingly cheerful types, greeting each new day with a smile (yuk). If we can all manage to be something between these two extremes, we'll be ok.

So remember, there's no reason why Part Two of your life can't be even more interesting than Part One. For one thing, there is great joy to be had in just not caring as much any more. Life for young women can be such an exhausting round of self-doubt and worries about the future: will you ever find someone to love you? Will kids be part of the picture? And what about your career? But once you've hit fifty, most of those questions will have been answered and you can concentrate on making the most of the cards fate has dealt you.

In any case, being menopausal doesn't mean you're old. This is the middle bit. This is #metime. You have years ahead of you, and yes, bits of it are tricky, but seriously, I'd much rather be my age than twenty-two again!

C

CARB LOADING

'Once upon a time, when I was in my early twenties, I was anorexic. People look at me now as if to say, "I didn't know you could recover that well".' **JE**

Whether you like it or not, the menopause can be pretty brutal in terms of what it can do to your body.

Let's start with weight. In my experience, a woman's metabolism is affected by her hormones and as they start to misbehave, merely standing outside a fish-and-chip shop inhaling the aroma of hot batter and vinegar is enough to burst the zip on your jeans.

It's not enough to make us hot and bothered, oh no – just when we need a little bit of help around the gut, Mother Nature plays her cruellest trick. She goes and adds fat into the mix. Oh great, the triple whammy: hot, bothered and fat.

Of course, it would be fine if this weight was evenly distributed around our entire bodies. An extra couple of millimetres all over wouldn't be too traumatic. But for some reason, all the weight piles on in spuddy lumps in just a few specific areas.

Firstly, it gathers around the gut – an effect colloquially known as the muffin top, whereby, basically, we become bulgy around the middle. Weirdly, there is a moment when you look in the mirror and for a second you are exactly the same Humpty-Dumpty shape that you were when you were pregnant back in the day.

Most women will also find they will go up a couple of bra sizes, which is fine if you've been dealt a small rack to begin with, but not so great if you've always been well endowed and now feel like you're carrying a couple of albatrosses around your neck on a daily basis. For me, having always been mean-bosomed, it's been quite nice to develop a proper pair of jugs, and these days I think they're one of my better features.

Great knockers are one thing, but there seems little point in the arrival of a sudden mass of back fat which accompanies the menopause like a large, unwanted rucksack. Back fat is sneaky. It creeps up on you and it's only when you are in one of those hideously cruel mirrored changing rooms that you realize you have deep, deep creases of folded fat around the back of your body.

The whole back fat thing really confuses me. Back fat belongs on camels. It's to keep them going during long walks through the desert when they can feed off their humps. Think how much more pleasurable having back fat would be if it was of any practical use – if it was made up of hummus, say, and could be squeezed on to pitta bread on a long walk.

And it's not just back fat. Great big dollops of unnecessary flesh will unexpectedly start bursting out in the oddest places. Suddenly, your calves are as meaty as a rugby player's and your knees are the size of giant turnips. Your ankles swell and your thighs gain six inches in circumference. There is something a bit Incredible Hulk-ish about the menopause and it can be bewildering.

There seems to be no real practical advantages to menopausal weight gain, aside from standing on the foot of someone you really dislike and seeing them wince in pain. But apart from that? No, sorry, can't think of anything else.

The problem with putting on weight is that people will automatically assume that you will want to lose it, and even if you do, it's really annoying that this assumption is so widespread. Everyone, from your mother to the ads that pop up without invitation on your Instagram account, will presume that your one abiding ambition is to get through the menopause without putting on an ounce.

Well, good luck with that, ladies, because there are many reasons why we lard up a bit at this time of life and not all of them are our fault:

- **Metabolism** It's been medically proven that our metabolism does slow down and because our bodies are confused, they tend to hold on to the fat thinking that, like animals, we might need it, possibly for a really cold winter.
- **Stress** I reckon 100 per cent of menopausal women suffer from stress, which produces the hormone cortisol (well known for its association with fight or flight) and cortisol is a bugger for piling on the pounds around your middle.
- **Poor sleep** This is also linked to weight gain. I read it on the Internet, so it must be true. If you don't believe me, Google it.
- **Increased insulin resistance** Yet another age-/menopause-related symptom which can make losing weight even harder (see what we're up against, girls?). What's more, for some reason, fat storage moves to our tummies during the menopause, which can increase our risk of type 2 diabetes and heart disease. Oh, great.
- **Comfort eating** Sometimes during the menopause things can get on top of us and all we're good for is lying on the sofa with a tin of biscuits, binge-watching *RuPaul's Drag Race*. Comfort

eating is one of the main causes of menopausal weight gain, we know this, we're not thick, but sometimes we can be very pig-headed and incredibly resistant to advice. Especially from women's magazines, most of which can't seem to make up their minds whether we should love ourselves, curves and all, or despise every ounce that takes us over nine stone.

So if you are quite happy carrying a few extra pounds, enjoy being able to keep toffees down your cleavage for the first time in your life and don't mind wobbling all over like a monster lady Jelly Baby when you try and trot for the bus, then fine.

However, if you do mind, it's time to take action because if you moan about getting fat, but refuse to do anything about it, you are just going to perpetuate a cycle of self-loathing. So unless you want to be fat for life, sadly the menopause is the time to start tweaking what you eat and drink.

ALCOHOL

Unfortunately, the biggest calorie saving you can make should you be into playing the weight-loss game is to give up the booze, or at least reduce your units.

To be honest, most middle-aged women find themselves cutting down on their units quite naturally, because there is something about the menopause that means drinking over your limit, even by the tiniest sip, will result in a crippling hangover during which you have to hold on to the kitchen surfaces whilst attempting to make a cup of tea in the morning. Menopausal hangovers are the very worst. Take a normal hangover and magnify it x 1,000 and you're getting close. Let's just say that things like opening a tin of cat food and spooning jellied chunks of rabbit into a plastic bowl will have you heaving over the sink for a good half hour.

Gradually, you realize this is not a virus. You can no longer drink like a one-woman hen night, and swigging from a bottle of rosé before going down the tequila-shots route will make you wish you were dead in the morning.

Here are the simple rules of menopausal drinking:

- Drink one glass of really nice, posh wine rather than three glasses of cheap rubbish.
- Do not drink on public transport. You will not look like you're having fun, you will look like you've got a problem (long-distance, intercity train journeys are obviously an exception to this rule).
- Do not drink during the day. You will fall asleep for the entire afternoon.
- Do not drink and shop; this is when expensive mistakes are made and you will lose the receipts.
- Do not drink Pimm's to refresh yourself on a hot day – not unless you fancy falling into a flowerbed mid-afternoon.

On the other hand, DO drink:

- if you don't care what anyone thinks about you and anyway you quite fancy telling the same story over and over and over again until you can't remember how it ends and you think you might die of hiccupping.

FOOD

Alas, unless you are going to get a gang of menopausal women together and play hockey/netball three times a week, you can no longer eat what you like without your knickers feeling the strain.

You don't need me to advise you about what you should eat as a menopausal woman, not when every other bugger on the planet is sticking their nose in (including your mate smug Sandra who still puts on her wedding dress now and again just to check she's the same weight as she was thirty years ago – grrrr).

All of us are bombarded with healthy-eating advice whatever our age and size, so I'm going to keep this quite general.

We all know it's pretty vital at this time to adopt a healthy-eating regime, but this should never be confused with a diet. Diets are all about self-denial, whilst healthy eating is all about allowing yourself the pleasure of eating well-cooked good food three times a day.

However, it's also about not sabotaging those three healthy meals with a load of ridiculous snacks in between. There's no point making yourself poached eggs for breakfast, a nice salad for lunch and steamed fish with green veg for supper if you're going to gobble six doughnuts and a tub of Ben & Jerry's on the side. If we're going to be sensible, then we'll do as we're told. To start with, cut down on the snacks: do we really need those sweets, biscuits, sausage rolls? Really? If the answer's yes, then eat it. If the answer's no, have an apple instead.

Of course, it's so much harder to practise what everyone preaches, when food is so bound up with emotions, self-esteem, boredom, habit and needing little treats. So don't beat yourself up if you occasionally have a greed frenzy, but don't expect incredible results if you don't try.

And when I say try, I don't mean try *too* hard. Be sensible. Personally, I'm very anti intermittent fasting, meaning the 5/2 regime, for example, when you eat normally for five days a week but fast for two. It works for some people, but I tend to get migraines if I starve myself and it's hard to look great even in a pair of size ten jeans if you're staggering around throwing up.

Crash diets are really bad for women of our age. Very low-calorie diets may result in short-term weight loss, but research shows that their impact on muscle mass and metabolic rate will make keeping that weight off even harder.

And the worst thing you can do is restrict your calories to the point where the resulting decrease in muscle mass could lead to bone loss, increasing your chances of osteoporosis.

So don't go mad and start living on grapefruit and boiled eggs like our mums did back in the 1970s. You can make small but significant changes to your diet without it feeling like a punishment.

- These days, it's all about dietary restraint rather than restriction. For example, watch your portion sizes, don't stray into Desperate Dan territory and resist going back for seconds. Remember, if you resist seconds of supper you've got a ready-made lunch waiting for you tomorrow – save time, save money, save calories, win, win, win.
- Cut down on bread by having an open sandwich loaded up with salad stuff (tricky on the move, but great for lunches at home).

- Make your own veggie soup, even if it's boring old carrot and coriander. A small mugful will take the edge off your appetite and make a healthy salad meal feel a great deal more filling. Add an apple after and, bingo, that's a three-course feast.
- Experiment with veg. Some of us have got a bit stuck in our ways, but the young people are veg mad. If you don't like cauliflower, try roasting it and BTW, that new fangled harissa spice adds a bit of zing to loads of things.

You don't need to go completely vegan to experiment with vegan recipes; no one's going to report you to the police if you pop a piece of grilled chicken on the side. And don't forget fish; it's easier to cook than you might think (says me who once nearly fainted over a mackerel that was in the process of being gutted) – a decent fishmonger will help you out on which varieties to buy and how to cook them.

Remember, for interesting recipes that don't need to hurt your purse, the Internet is your friend.

We all know the rules, lean meat, green leafy veg, oily fish, pulses, grains and plenty of fresh fruit. Oh and porridge, the dullest thing you can put in your mouth (unless, of course, you've ever sucked off Tim Henman*), but apparently, it can help you live till you're a hundred – not that you'd want to live till you were a hundred. Not if it meant eating porridge every day.

As someone who never learned to cook until I was menopausal, may I just say that I'm now a complete convert to getting my own pans out. Ok, it's a bore having to do all that washing up, but I do think we're better off having a break from processed food and all

---

* Apologies, old joke (and totally untrue, by the way. I've never sucked off Tim Henman, for the record), but it still makes me laugh.

those E numbers once in a while. Cooking for yourself is oddly therapeutic, but if, like me, you've remained a novice right up until you hit your fifties, don't try and run before you can walk. Jamie Oliver's *5 Ingredients* is the book that eventually gave me cooking confidence. Listen, if I can do it, anyone can, and I promise the results are cheaper, healthier and more satisfying on every level.

PS If you eat meat, make sure you've got chicken thighs on your shopping list. They're low fat, one of the cheapest cuts on the meat counter and incredibly versatile – seriously, you can do anything with them: marinate, stir-fry, stuff, curry, risotto, casserole, tagine. If you need any more ideas, just go online. There's a world of chicken thigh recipes out there.

Here's one of my store-cupboard stand-bys that I have adapted from a recipe I found online – it's called Very Sticky Summer Thighs, which is a phrase I think all menopausal women can sympathize with.

VERY STICKY SUMMER CHICKEN THIGHS

Serves 4 / 5 depending on greediness

Ingredients

a couple of garlic cloves, crushed

2 lemons

2 tbsp clear runny honey plus a little extra to add at the last minute

1 tbsp Worcestershire sauce

2 good teasp. grainy mustard, to taste

10 boneless chicken thighs, skin on or off

sea salt and a few twists of black pepper, to taste

Method

Crush the garlic.

Squeeze the juice from the two lemons, fishing out any pips. Add the honey, Worcestershire sauce and the mustard and mix thoroughly. Add the garlic, salt and pepper, and mix again.

Place the chicken thighs in an oven-proof dish, making sure they do not overlap. Pour the marinade over the chicken and rub in. Leave in the fridge to marinate for at least 1 hour.

Add a thin glazing of honey over the thighs and place in a preheated oven at 200°C (fan; a little higher for a conventional oven) and cook for 45 minutes, turning halfway through.

I haven't mentioned cake, chocolate, cheese or crisps in this chapter. Listen, I don't want to trigger a binge, but we all know these are the things we must only eat either when nothing else will do, or it would be rude not to.

Personally, I'm not fussed about cake and I haven't eaten chocolate in over forty years, but my biggest downfalls are crisps and cheese. The last time I got drunk, I woke up in a hotel room convinced my arm was in a plaster cast. Once I'd shed some light on the situation, however, I realized I'd passed out up to my elbow in a tube of Pringles. Sometimes I have no willpower.

As for my cheese habit, it's not helped by my management signing me up for a cheese club membership last Xmas. Every month a large consignment of different posh cheeses arrives at my door and every month I try and give at least half of it away, donating it to friends and neighbours. I don't want to, but if it's in my fridge, I'll eat it.

Oh, God, even typing this is making me want to eat some cheese. Aarghhhh – there's nothing quite like cheese is there? You can cut up your strips of snacking veg crudités and keep them handy but a stick of celery ain't never gonna compete with a great big wodge of bursting-out-of-its-rind brie.

Cheese is my chocolate. We all have something that we find difficult to resist and for me, it's cheese and Keanu Reeves. Oooh, imagine a life-size Keanu Reeves made out of cheese . . .

Popcorn: that's the answer to snacking. Plain salt popcorn is only around a hundred calories a bag. And rice cakes. They're good too. Spread 'em with smashed avo/banana or low-fat cream cheese or cottage cheese and Marmite.

Finally, nuts and seeds nuts are good for you, but only if you can stop at one small handful. Try not to con yourself into thinking a jumbo bag of dry-roasted peanuts is a daily necessity.

And almonds are good for the brain, apparently (unfortunately, they do not need to be sugar coated).

Good luck, everyone. And remember, if willpower fails, then fuck it. You're invisible now anyway, so who cares if you put on another five stone!

D

DOGS AND OTHER DISTRACTIONS

'Sometimes you just want something to cuddle. Hot-water bottles are good, but they never look particularly pleased to see you.' **JE**

A great number of women my age are very grandchild broody. If they haven't got one already, they're looking into prams, thinking, Ah, sweet, I want one of those; but only part-time, maybe for a couple of hours every other week.

I'm still not at that stage. I'm the kind of woman who goes on holidays and dreads ending up in the room next door to a six-month-old squawker. But whilst I don't get remotely broody over babies, show me a miniature smooth-haired dachshund and it's all I can do not to attempt a dog snatch.

I never had a pet of my own as a child. When I was very young my father was in the army, which meant we moved around and lived abroad for a number of years. I can't remember actually asking for a pet either (mind you, I never asked for a younger brother and one of those arrived, dammit). In truth, I was scared of dogs thanks to a neighbourhood Alsatian that stalked our strasse when we lived in Berlin and I've never really given cats the time of day.

I probably didn't obsess over the lack of a pet in my life at the time because most of my mates came from military families and they didn't have pets either. People don't tend to commit to dogs when they're not sure where their next posting will be, and back then there was no such thing as a pet passport. In any case, we lived in army quarters and animals were strictly verboten.

Things changed when my father left the army and we settled in the north of England where I finished off my primary education at a local state school and where some of my new friends did have pets. I remember Carolyn Reynolds' fat yellow Labrador who used to lick the knives and forks whenever it waddled past their open dishwasher, which used to make me feel a bit sick, to be quite honest.

Then, my friend Jane Davey got some rabbits and went rabbit mad, training them to leap over jumps in the back garden (jumps that only a year before we'd been jumping over ourselves as we pretended to be horses). I wasn't much interested in Jane's rabbits (they might have been hares) or her tortoise or her creepy stick insects.

My pet pilot light remained unignited, even years later when my parents bought my much younger brother a Westie called Humphrey. I took very little notice of it, ditto his boring bunnies and a couple of love birds, one of whom was called Doris.

Even though we now officially had pets, none of them belonged to me. In fact, as a kid, the only animal I rushed to check up on was a life-size terracotta stone rabbit that perched amongst my grandparents' rockery in Poulton-le-Fylde. For some reason, this inanimate object meant rather a lot to me and I can't believe that my sister now has possession of the thing, badly chipped ears and all.

As the years passed by and I left home and lived in bedsits before coming to London and meeting the man who is still my partner, the subject of pets never came up. He was a cat lover with asthma;

I was disinterested. Maybe we had a fairground fish for a while, but nothing else until we moved into a house with a garden and our daughter started begging for something furry. It was either that or a younger sibling and that wasn't going to happen. Phoebe was probably about seven when we bought her a rabbit from the kind of pet shop that is no longer allowed to exist. Remember? They used to be on every high street – all sorts of animals kept in stupidly small cages, wee-wee sawdust all over the shop floor and at the back under strange lighting there was always a tankful of snakes giving the gerbils on the opposite shelf evils. Anyway, Flopsy was a sweet white and beige lop-eared beauty – an incredibly photogenic and good-natured creature, who lived for a short while in a hutch outside the back door. When I say a short time, I mean . . . well, foxes . . . south London and all that; anyway, I presume it was a fox – all I know is that it disappeared one day, no trace of blood, no nothing, just gone.

We bought Phoebe a hamster after that which, for safety's sake, lived in her bedroom, even though the sound of it running around on its wheel at night drove us mad. The hamster was quite sweet, but he kept unsociable hours and anyway he died. Only we thought he was hibernating, so that was all rather unfortunate because Phoebe's bedroom was really stinking before we realized, so that was a difficult Christmas.

Since then nothing. No pets, no craving for a pet. We lived a pet-free existence without ever realizing something might be missing.

Back up north, at my parents' place, Humphrey the Westie got dementia, started pissing in my mum's wardrobe and was put down. By this point both my adult siblings had dogs in the house: my sister bought my nephew a bad-tempered schnauzer who lived for fourteen furious years before the vet put him out of his barking misery, whilst my brother had a beloved blue whippet, who eventually succumbed to lymphoma and was put down the week my nephew and niece embarked on their finals and A levels respectively.

I could have said 'I told you so', but didn't (well, I did but very quietly under my breath). Because I've always had this theory that if you buy a child a dog for his/her seventh birthday, sod's law says it will die on the eve of his/her finals. Do the maths – most dogs live on average for about fourteen years: $14 + 7 = 21$. How old are most kids when they're doing their finals? I rest my case. Sadly for my nephew Gabriel this mathematical prophecy came true, and I doubt he was the only one going into an exam room with a heavy heart. In fact, I very much feel all pet-bereaved finalists should be awarded an extra ten points in any subsequent exams.

So, after all that, what I'm trying to say, in rather a long-winded way, is that a dog might be the answer to many menopausal women's misery. Obviously, each menopausal woman is different from the next, but one of the things we all share is the need for a little bit of unconditional love.

Ok, so some of us are lucky to have a partner knocking around, but much as I love Geof, I don't want him sitting on my lap on the sofa.

Many of us have children too, and God knows we love them, but sadly (or not, see Chapter E for Empty Nest) for many menopausal women they've flown the coop and when they do come home, they don't want to snuggle up next to you having their tummies rubbed. But doggies don't mind this kind of treatment. Doggies like getting up on sofas they're not supposed to sit on and are quite happy to loll around being tickled and stroked.

I'm thinking every menopausal woman should be offered a dog on the National Health. I have never felt so canine broody in all my life, and I certainly never thought as long and hard about having a baby as I have about a dog. Although, to be fair, I got pregnant completely by accident and that's not going to happen with a dog.

Of course, when I say I want a dog, there are provisos.

What I really want is a dog who's already been trained not to chew anything expensive and not to shit or piss indoors.

I don't really want a dog who knocks things over either. My brother's blue whippet could walk into an antique shop without anyone flinching; he was the most delicate of dogs with only the gentlest wag in his tail, incapable of bumping into anything – but he was also too thin-skinned to walk near a barb-wire fence and I need something a little more boisterous and silly.

However, I don't want a dog who needs a great deal of walking, so something with a shortish leg to match mine is what I'm after.

Fortunately for all wannabe dog owners, the Internet is on hand to feed our craving. I've been spending a great deal of time doing 'Which dog would suit you?' quizzes online – but they keep coming back with French bulldogs, and I'm really sorry but I don't want anything that breathes louder than the old man. I'm not having two snorers in the house.

Plus, my mate Podcast Judith was right when she asked if these quizzes mention turd size and regularity. Because, let's be honest, that's got to enter into the equation when it comes to choosing a dog. I don't want anything that's going to require a bin liner rather than a doggie bag.

So what I really want in my new best friend is a lazy, slightly constipated mutt who doesn't like the taste of leather or furniture, but does like freshening his/her breath with peppermints and pops out the occasional very small, dried turd – the kind you could sweep or hoover away.

Currently, I've narrowed my puppy obsession down to a final three: a dachshund, a Bedlington and a miniature Airedale. I also like poodles but the old man thinks he might be suspected of cottaging if he took a poodle to our local park. Secretly, I know that somewhere out there a little black and tan dachshund is waiting for me to come and take him home.

Not all of us can have pets. There are allergies, work commitments and landlords to consider and we shouldn't rush into these decisions.

On the other hand . . . I do want a doggie.

OTHER DISTRACTIONS

If a dog or any pet is a no-no, then there are other things us menopausal madams can do to improve our lives.

For one thing, there are dog-loaning schemes in many areas now. There's one called BorrowMyDoggy, which basically does what it says on the tin: dog owners who are struggling to give their pooch enough exercise or attention for whatever reason – be it work or health or family problems – are matched up with would-be walkers/strokers/playmates. This is the ideal solution for those who would like a dog but can't house one full time. Snooping around the website, it seems that both dog owners and borrowers are benefiting not only from bonding with the dog but with the owners too.

But it's not just pets that need affection. My friend Anneka Rice (jumpsuit, blonde, ridiculously youthful, all-round good egg and most excellent painter) swears by a scheme in her neighbourhood which matches up people who have a bit of spare time with the very elderly. Anneka regularly meets up with several women in their eighties, taking them on jaunts, giving them lifts and afternoon tea treats. But mostly it's about talking, and she is absolutely insistent that she is the one who gets the most out of it. Age UK operate similar schemes around the country, if you're interested.

Volunteering is something that for most of us exists in a hazy 'one-day-I'll-get-round-to-it' kind of way, but for a lot of people it's something they do, week in week out. They drive minibuses and visit the elderly, they shop and deliver meals, they change light bulbs and do small jobs around the house. Sometimes all people want is a picture hung up somewhere they can see it.

How you get the most out of your life as a menopausal woman is entirely up to you. What fulfils one of us might leave another cold. But life doesn't stop just because all your eggs are gone – my sister is doing a part-time history degree, my friend Podcast Judith has trained as a grief counsellor, my mum knows someone who reads the papers for her local blind community, a retired teacher from my daughter's old school is now qualified to comfort prem babies at King's, a neighbour of mine helps kids who are struggling to read gain confidence at the local primary . . .

And even if you can't commit to a regular role, there are other ways to feel a bit better about yourself simply by helping other people. Knit squares for blankets, sign up for that charity walk, donate a fundraising cake, talk to the woman who lives on her own over the road – you don't have to cross the threshold, but even waving and smiling can give both of you a bit of a lift.

If there's one thing the menopause has taught me, it's that we all need to be kinder: kinder to other people and kinder to ourselves.

EMPTY NEST

'It's not until your children leave home that you realize quite how long a packet of cereal can last.' **JE**

Not every menopausal woman has children, so I'm sorry if this chapter is annoying. That said, I don't think you need to have children to experience the empty nest, so bear with me here.

Missing a much-loved pet can be just as painful, but for those of us who happened to have skin babies, losing them to adulthood can be a really tricky period of transition and it tends to happen at a time when you feel you are losing just about everything else – your looks, your figure, your marbles – so when the kids bugger off too, it can feel a little bit 'last straw'.

It doesn't matter if you have one child or fifteen, the empty nest is still 'a thing'. Of course, the experience is a lot easier if you can't stand your children's guts and finally getting rid of them is a cause for much celebration. But most of us are pretty fond of the fruit of our loins and seeing them leave home can be a traumatic business.

So to soften the blow, I've written an 'Empty Nest – Reasons to be Grateful' checklist:

Older and Wider

1. For the first time since you gave birth, you will start sleeping through the night (unless your bladder is as weak as mine), especially at the weekends. You will no longer spend the wee hours of Saturday and Sunday morning convinced the next time the phone goes it's going to be the police informing you that your presence is required at the station/hospital/morgue.

2. You will no longer have to remain sober on Friday and Saturday nights in case you need to get the car out and rescue anyone who went to a party somewhere beyond the reach of public transport and wants to come home because their 'tummy hurts'.

3. Your food will go so much further – especially if you are the parent of boys. (Boys eat a shocking amount of food; I've seen teenage boys reach in the fridge for a snack and inhale whole tubs of hummus, complete with entire packs of pitta bread and a side tube of Pringles, all washed down with a litre-bottle of juice – and not the cheap concentrate, the good stuff that *you* drink by the thimbleful at breakfast because it's so expensive. Teenage boys are nothing but giant locusts in great big smelly trainers.)

4. You will no longer be subjected to the stench of said trainers. Hooray, your house will no longer smell like a cheesemonger's – a cheesemonger's where a rat curled up and died in the Stilton. No, your house will smell normal. It might take some time, but eventually you will walk in one day and you won't feel like throwing up at the pong.

5. Your electricity bills will plummet, particularly if you have children of the female persuasion – because once they've gone, you can readjust your thermostat to something a little

more Ipswich than Ibitha. For some reason, young women are incapable of keeping warm via a nice, thick woolly jumper. They much prefer to wander around in their vest and knickers with every radiator turned up as high as possible. As for their trigger-happy immersion-heater habits – don't get me started.

6. You will have unlimited access to the bathroom and your towels will be dry because they've been returned to the towel rail. Sheets and pillowcases will no longer be heavily stained with hair dye/foundation/tears. Whoop, those hysterical nut jobs with their weeping and wailing and door slamming have gone. What's that you can hear? That's called silence – cherish it.

7. That nice fat bundle of notes that was in your purse at the beginning of the week is still there (more or less) at the end of it because no one has tapped you for a couple of quid/a tenner/twenty, Mum, and I promise I'll pay it back. Now, with any luck you should have enough spending money left over for a really nice bottle of wine or a takeaway – or possibly both.

8. The remote control is yours, all yours (unless you have a partner, in which case I suggest you work out a rota). The main thing is that you will be able to watch your programmes in peace from now on. There won't be any silly, dramatic yawning during *Sewing Bee* or puke noises when little babies are born during *Call the Midwife*. From now on you can watch all the cooking, craft, little-babies-being-born programmes. Plus, there will be space on the sofa to put your feet up. Win, win.

9. Your laundry basket will be mostly empty. In fact, some days you won't actually have to bother putting a wash on. This will feel like being reborn.

10. There is no longer an empty Marmite jar in the cupboard, because the person who scraped the last remnants will have rinsed it out, put it in the recycling and made a note to buy more. Actually, sod it – the person who likes Marmite doesn't live in the house any more, so you don't have to buy another jar of the disgusting stuff ever again; if they want Marmite when they come and visit, then they can jolly well bring their own.

11. There will be no more sticky finger or massive great hand prints on your stainless-steel fridge freezer, because unlike some people, you learned years ago how to open it by its HANDLE.

12. Your phone charger will always be where you left it. It won't be 'at Katy's because I accidentally took it round there and left it and now she's gone to Guadeloupe'.

13. You won't have to retune your impossibly complicated digital radio back to Radio 4 after someone's twiddled the knobs around to some mad dance station and set the volume so high that you have a small heart attack when you first turn it on.

14. Your cashmere scarf will be in your drawer and not on the back seat of the 176 night bus.

15. You won't have to worry that those sounds emanating from his/her bedroom might be sex noises.

On the downside, you will keep wasting your money on food which no one eats, until there are great hummus pots of fur clogging up your fridge.

You could, of course, clear all this rubbish out, fill your shelves with miso and umami paste and start cooking experimental dinners which you can eat on your knees in front of all those telly programmes you always wanted to watch but never could because for some reason you always caved into the kids and what they wanted to watch.

But weirdly, you don't have much of an appetite any more.

RECLAIMING SPACE

When your children first leave home you will enter a period of semi-mourning. This will involve drooping around the house, sitting on the ends of their beds, sniffing their dressing gowns and crying. This is when you will find a packet of fags in your child's dressing-gown pocket, even though they swore blind to you they didn't smoke.

At this point it's very important not to start snooping. This is tough on middle-aged women. The female of the species is a born snooper and with age it just gets worse. However, if you start now, when you are at your most vulnerable, you will only find things that upset you. I once found a diary of my daughter's, written when she was eight, describing how annoying I was on a trip to Venice and how I kept almost spoiling the holiday by being 'weird and selfish'. So let that be a lesson to you. Ever since I read those passages I have never gone near any of my daughter's diaries, despite the fact that I would quite like concrete proof that she lost her virginity on a certain date back in 2006 (there was something about her face the next day – a kind of smugness I'd never seen before). But even though I know where they are, I wouldn't even peek, having learned that children's diaries are likely to go off like a small bomb in your face.

For months or even years (ten in our case) you will not touch their bedroom. After all, what if they need to come home? We all have traumatic memories of our parents redecorating and coming home to find that our wardrobe is no longer covered in lipstick kisses and Gallery Five stickers. The soppier you are about your children, the longer you will leave their bedroom in some kind of shrine-like state. Even when my daughter turned thirty and was living with her boyfriend in New Cross, her teenage bedroom remained *circa* 2005, complete with boxes of Barbies and Polly Pockets. (Try as I might, I cannot get rid of the Polly Pockets. Have you seen them? Aw . . . they have such sweet faces and they live in tiny shell-shaped houses and little palaces and some of them move on tiny magnets under their feet.)

My friend Podcast Judith, whose daughter recently got married, has got the 'what-to-do-with-the-bedroom' bug really bad. As she says, her daughter is now a married woman, she is a Mrs – surely, if ever there's a time to reclaim the bedroom it's when they're married off, and yet she's still finding excuses to 'leave it for the time being'.

Back at our house, my partner mumbles about the waste of space, the good light that floods into Phoebe's bedroom, its attic studio potential. And yes, there's a big part of me that can easily imagine a couple of easels permanently set up, oil paints out, stinking to high heaven and even a table with a sewing machine on it (where has this fantasy come from?). But there's still a part that can't make the Polly Pockets homeless. Not yet. Maybe in a couple of years.

LOOKING FORWARD

As long as your child hasn't moved continent, you can still see them (and even if they have moved continent, there's always Skype).

Of course, in our wildest dreams, what we really want our children to do is make the transition into adulthood and complete independence as smoothly as possible, with a career that makes them happy (solvent) and even a nice, supportive partner (preferably a really practical one who will do lots of little jobs around your house, free of charge).

We all have secret fantasies about them picking us up in their fancy car (which they can suddenly drive, despite having failed their test nine times whilst living under our roof) and taking us back to their place (about thirty minutes away is ideal) for a slap-up lunch (on a properly laid table) before driving us home. The reality is more likely to be a couple of bus rides to somewhere a bit disappointing and a massive row which is all your fault because you were daft enough to criticize the roller blind in their bathroom.

Sometimes it's hard to accept your children are adults now and they are allowed to make their own decisions. You are no longer the puppet meister, so if they decide to keep newts, tattoo their legs and dye their hair green, it's got nothing to do with you.

This is also the stage of life when you will meet other mothers around the same age as you who will want to bang on about how successful their children are, how established their careers, how well paid, how secure and settled . . . But as all of us know, life is very complicated and in a few years' time those same women might be avoiding you like the plague because it's all come horribly unravelled. No one has it easy all the time.

Older and Wider

Letting your kids go is hard work. Sometimes you've got to sit back and watch them make terrible mistakes (and not just about carpets and roller blinds) without saying a word. Whatever you do, try not to fan the flames of whatever relationship/work/money crisis they're having. Because the last thing you want them to do is run home to Mummy – not when you've finally got the house exactly how you like it.

After all, the nest might be empty, but you're no longer tripping over discarded shoes and other assorted crap. Silver linings, ladies.

FRESH AIR

'When I was young, I hated going for walks. Left/right, left/ right, plod, plod, plod in a great big circle until you were allowed to get back in the car. What was the point in all that? But now . . .' **JE**

When you're feeling a little bit GRRRrrrrrrrrr or even a lot GRRR-rrrrrrrr and nothing else is working, try walking. Try leaving the house and getting a bit of fresh air into your lungs.

I can hardly believe I wrote that!

Because, as a younger, chain-smoking dirty stop-in, I was never one for fresh air. There was nothing I enjoyed more than sitting writing in my sliver of a study, with a litre bottle of Diet Coke and a brimming ashtray by my side. I was so disinterested in the great outdoors that entire train journeys could pass by without me bothering to look out of the window. I barely noticed the change in seasons. My mother would phone and say, 'Did it rain today?' and I wouldn't have a clue. My world was very small: there was my work, me and the mirror.

All that has changed since the menopause.

Don't get me wrong. I'm still not one for long rambles across vast open spaces. I'm a lazy cow, and the idea of a really good, long walk terrifies the living daylights out of me. For starters, what do you mean by a long walk? For me, a walk is too long if I can't see a cafe out of the corner of my eye.

That said, even the biggest fresh air phobe will come to realize that, now and again, the only thing that is going to make you feel better is to put your shoes and coat on and physically leave the house.

Sometimes we need to 'blow the cobwebs away' as my mother (and probably every other mother) would say.

Obviously, lots of menopausal women walk as part of their daily commute. Some are lucky enough to have dogs, but for those of us who are dog free and work from home (and as a consequence barely ever get out of their pyjamas), sometimes you forget that a bit of fresh air can make all the difference.

And even if you do walk as part of your daily routine, you can always mix it up a bit: walk to the next bus stop rather than the one nearest to your front door, go the other way around to the Tube or the train station, try a different park. Take deep breaths in and out and swing your arms. Walk even if you have nowhere to go. Walk even if you don't want to – dare yourself to walk around the block. Because even if you do nothing else all day, you will have been outside, and this is better than not going outside. Gradually, if you make yourself go for a walk every day, you might even start looking forward to it – you might make your walks longer, and eventually you will start noticing things like trees. Obviously, noticing trees is loads easier if you live in the countryside where they are ten a penny. But even in the middle of London there are more trees than you might imagine. It's not all burned-out cars and incident tape, you know.

Now trees can be a bit of a bind if you suffer from hay fever, but even if you are red-eyed and sneezing, it's incredible to see what

Mother Nature can do. Forget Lady Gaga and her umpteen outfit changes for the Met gala ball – Mother Nature will show you tricks and transformations that will make your jaw drop.

Because Nature never stops and never gives up. She gives us snowdrops in February, tulips and daffodils in March, cherry blossom in April, wisteria in May, and on she goes throughout the year treating us to all sorts of goodies, magnolias, catkins and bluebells, frogspawn, hollyhocks and foxgloves . . . Nature will creep out from between the cracks of tarmacked car parks and run riot along the side of train tracks. She can survive anything – and so can we.

Take it from yours truly, reconnecting with Nature can really help to rebalance your moods.

Of course, not everyone can just go for a walk. Many menopausal women are not only dealing with the big M but with illnesses and other debilitating physical conditions as well. So for those who struggle to get out, even looking out of the window and really watching what's going on outside can help. You don't need much of a garden to notice some activity; mine's minute, but every day, as long as I put out some bread, we get magpies and blackbirds and fat pigeons and blue tits and squirrels – and this is in south London. Yes, I've got sirens and cop cars and ambulances belting past my house on a daily basis, but around the back, Nature is doing her best.

The great thing about fresh air is that it's free. It feels great against the skin and it might even make your eyes sparkle – and ok, so you might work up a bit of an appetite, but as long as you've been for a walk, then why not have that hot chocolate/burned sausage that's been lying under the grill since last night. You deserve it, lady.

Getting in touch with Nature, be it on a walk or even watching a wildlife programme, can be an incredible comfort when your life seems to have been turned upside down by your own body. Because it's not just you that is undergoing weird stuff. Just watch what happens to a caterpillar – one day, the menopause will be over and we will all emerge like butterflies (hmmm, might be stretching this metaphor slightly, considering by the time the menopause has done for us, we're twelve stone of fallen arches, but you know what I mean). Nature is all about change; it's also about optimism, as anyone who has ever grown a sunflower from a single seed will know. Which brings me to . . .

. . . GARDENING

This is a great hobby,

a. if you have a garden, and
b. if you have a pair of knees that don't scream in agony every time you get down on them.

Personally, as I've said, I don't have much of a garden, but I do have a huge, very squishy pair of knees, which look like they belong to a rugby player who has fallen many times. However, despite having the knees for it, I don't have the fingers – gardening is not my special thing, although that's not to say I don't appreciate it. And I love other people's gardens (particularly if they have a greenhouse that smells of olden-days tomatoes, just like my grandfather's did) and some of my favourite Instagram accounts are those of professional flower growers (@donsdahliasetc and @holkerhall for example).

So even though I know I'm never going to give Percy Thrower a run for his money (there's a ref that dates me), I did have a gardening epiphany last year when I was fifty-eight years old and on tour with *Grumpy Old Women to the Rescue*. We'd been gigging in Shrewsbury – one of my touring hot spots because, as far as I'm concerned, a city with a Singer Sewing machine repair shop is my kind of town. My fellow Grumpies on this tour were the indomitable chanteuse that is Dillie Keane and the extremely funny actress Lizzie Roper. Both are keen gardeners and had littered the back of the tour-mobile with seed catalogues, AKA 'gardening porn'.

It was Dillie who dropped it into the conversation: 'There's this, um, garden centre,' she growled. 'Pretty special, just roses. It's called the David Austin Rose Garden, not far away in Wolverhampton.' Which happened to be more or less en route to the next gig. So we took a small detour and, well . . . as we approached, I had a moment. There was a gap in a hedge and through it I saw a sea of roses – roses as far as the eye could see, miles of them, and that was just the surrounding fields. The garden centre itself is one of the wonders of the world. Obviously, it helped that it was a glorious June day (remember the summer of 2018) and we'd managed to hit peak rose season, bees hummed and, just like on bonfire night, there were involuntary cries of delight as people roamed the gardens, going 'Ooh' and 'Aaahhh', as they discovered a particular favourite and buried their noses deep into flowers like truffle pigs snuffling for scent. I have rarely seen so many happy people anywhere before. It was like a sort of heaven. And in Wolverhampton too!

We ate lunch (yes, of course, there's a cafe) with peacocks grazing around our feet and I went mad in the shop, after which I travelled to the next destination with a Desdemona rosebush clutched between my knees. Seriously, the only other time I cared so much for a passenger's safety was when I brought my newborn daughter home in the car for the very first time.

As it turned out, poor Desdemona had a twisted root and I mangled her rather badly as I grappled her from her pot in order to sit her in a bigger, better pot. Within a few days she had started to look a bit sorry for herself. No matter. I ordered three more healthy specimens, who arrived by post and bloomed non-stop until October. As I write this, in May, they are just starting to re-sprout (technical term?), and even Desdemona, in whom Dillie and Lizzie insisted I must never lose faith, has perked up and is looking a lovely bright green around the gills. Every morning I go out and sing to them, 'Hello, my lovely ladies, my lovely, lovely ladies' (I think I'm entitled to do this as tunelessly as I like, considering the kid next door does trumpet practice with the window open).

Potted rose bushes cost under thirty quid by post. They are the ideal gift for people like me who adore flowers but can't really be arsed to garden/have very limited space. Herbs in pots are also great for the tiny garden-owning non-gardener. There is something deliciously smug about adding your own herbs to a dish (though apparently, you should wash them first because cats don't know the difference between a pot of fresh herbs and a lavatory).

One last note for those who want to grow something from seed but haven't got any outdoor soil space – you can always harvest your own cress old-school style on a flannel in the airing cupboard.

HOW TO GROW CRESS AT HOME

You will need:

- a suitable (waterproof) container – something like an old margarine tub will do (washed out properly, mind)
- a piece of absorbent cloth/flannel or even some sturdy kitchen paper
- some cress seeds – available from garden centres or online.

Method:

- Fold the cloth over on itself a few times, so that it is quite thick and then cut it to a size that fits neatly into the container.
- Dampen the cloth and sprinkle the seeds on to it, forming a thick single layer, so that all the seeds are in contact with the damp cloth.
- Place the container in a warm, dark place (for instance, the bottom of your airing cupboard) and leave it there until the seeds begin to sprout. Germination will normally take about two days. EXCITING!
- When the seeds begin to sprout, move the container to a light location, such as a windowsill, stand back and let the magic happen. Check the moisture of the cloth frequently and add a little more water when necessary. In a few days you should have enough cress to make a delicious egg and cress sandwich.

Older and Wider

For those wanting to be a bit more extravagant, you can get these mad mushroom-growing kits online. Pricier than growing cress, but for under £20 you can grow your own pink oyster mushrooms in just a couple of weeks. I bought these kits as presents for my brother and sister one Christmas. My brother was delighted, but only because he was relieved it wasn't one of my paintings.

The Japanese are particularly keen on the idea that the great outdoors has healing properties; the belief system known as Shinto relies on a love of Nature. One of my great ambitions is to visit Japan during its famous blossom season, but failing that, I have to say East Dulwich in south London is a glorious place to be in April when the cherry blossom turns the world bright pink.

So Nature is good and the general consensus is that we all need to go outside and smell the roses now and then. And if there aren't any roses, have a sniff at something else, watch a squirrel eat a nut, actually take the time to watch those blue tits swing on your fat ball, collect conkers (kids don't want them any more because they don't make beeping noises). If you live in a city, take a bus to some green space, and if you are lucky enough to live anywhere near the sea, walk along a beach, pick up some interesting pebbles, listen to the waves and try to ignore that disgusting seagull pecking at a pool of vomit.

Mother Nature, eh! She's a hard mistress, as any menopausal woman will tell you. But seriously, sometimes it's useful to see what's going on in the world outside our own lives, and Nature is very good at reminding us that women have been going through what we are going through for centuries. Ageing is like the seasons – it's just part of the process.

G

GETTING YOUR SHIT TOGETHER

'Accepting that you're a proper adult is hard. In fact, every time I put petrol in my car, there's a bit of me that thinks, I can't believe they're letting me do this.' **JE**

The menopause can be a bit of a wake-up call. Rightly or wrongly, the mere fact that you can no longer have babies pushes you over an invisible line. Like it or not, you are not on the young side of the fence any more; you've crossed over into that nether world of three-quarter-length cargo trousers and shoes that look like Cornish pasties.

I'm talking metaphorically here, of course. There is nothing about the menopause that means you suddenly have to adopt a weird kind of 'Ramblers Association' uniform, despite the number of brochures that come through your door suggesting that you do. Resist the temptation, ladies. I'm fifty-nine and I still haven't got one of those padded sleeveless dog-walking gilets (although, occasionally, I do borrow one from my friend Podcast Judith who is sixty-four and has quite a collection of them in an array of togs and colours, purchased from various outlets, including that posh motorway service station near the Lake District (a Mecca for the menopausal, BTW)).

One of the most important things for a menopausal woman to

realize is that you are meat to advertising companies. Once they pick up on the fact that you have reached that certain time of life and they manage to get hold of your address, you will be bombarded with lifestyle catalogues. Contents will include anything from orthopaedic mattresses and hideous Celtic jewellery to hearing aids and Saga holidays. For pretty obvious reasons, quite a lot of holiday companies have cottoned on to the fact that the ultimate destination for the menopausal woman is a cruise around the Norwegian fjords, plus a chance to see the Northern Lights.

You've got to give these people some credit, it makes savvy business sense to offer millions of overheating women a nice, cool sailing trip around some chilly glaciers – just think, you could re-enact that iconic Kate Winslet *Titanic* moment and give it a menopausal twist by standing topless on the prow of the ship in below-zero temperatures. All those Mediterranean cruises and trips to the Caribbean can wait until you're out of the hot-flush years and fancy paying money to feel sweat trickling down your back again.

The darker side of crossing this invisible line is that suddenly you will start doing sums in your head. You will start wondering about how long you're going to live and how much money you are going to need. The trouble with these kinds of sums is that there is no one correct answer. None of us has a clue, guessing is ridiculous and at this point you will begin to regret not having the kind of job that gives you a pension.

Aaaargh, excuse me whilst I have a self-indulgent panic.

Yes, I might have worked in Australia and had more fun than you can shake a stick at in Iceland and Finland, but as I hurtle towards sixty, I wonder what it would have been like to have had a job that paid into a pension and gave me some kind of future security. But that's my problem to deal with (although I am toying with the idea of crowd-funding a pension pot).

All joking aside, it's pretty important around now to start acting your age and facing up to all that stuff you've been ignoring for years. Being irresponsible is kind of cute when you're young, but once you're middle-aged it's just reckless and selfish. This is the time to get your affairs in order. For example, I got married after thirty-five years of happily living in sin. This was on my accountant's advice – tax and death duties might not be the most romantic of reasons to tie the knot, but there's nothing romantic about the taxman laughing all the way to the bank, just because you couldn't be bothered to make it legal before you died.

Oh yes – and make a will. Over 8 million people over the age of fifty haven't done this. Seriously, it's not difficult. Just find your nearest friendly local solicitor and make an appointment. Not making a will is like leaving a massive pile of litter behind and no one will thank you for it.

I think that for many menopausal women, when you don't feel like you have much control over your own mind and body, it's really important to help yourself feel less chaotic in other ways. For me, this involves getting on top of things, doing some list-ticking-off and tidying up the house.

DECLUTTERING

The menopause is a reminder that you're over halfway through – do you really want to live the rest of your life like a teenager? Now is the time to take stock, because the alternative is to risk going full-on hoarder, turning into one of those old bats who has to tunnel through piles of newspaper to get from one room to the next.

You are not going to get any younger; the clock is not going to magically start reversing. So this is the time to decide how you want to live in the future.

The quickest way to start feeling more organized is to go around your house/flat and empty every single bin. This won't take long, but the benefits are huge. In literally minutes your place will look like it's had a spring clean.

Next, do you really need all that crap in your wardrobe? Mid-menopause I had a sudden revelation. I had seven pairs of size twelve jeans tucked away in case I ever got thin enough to wear them again. Basically, I had a decision to make: I was either going to try and get into those jeans or I was going to continue eating brie. Denim or brie? Brie won. I kept two pairs on the off chance and put the other five in the charity bag.

Try as I might though, I cannot go the full Kondo. Now for those who have been in prison over the past couple of years and have therefore missed out on the whole 2019 Kondo thing, let me briefly explain. Marie Kondo is the sweet Japanese woman who took over social media for a while with her YouTube videos on the art of Kondoing. (To Kondo is basically Japanese for 'tidying'.)

Marie's method is simple: if something doesn't 'spark joy', then get rid of it. And she demonstrates what she preaches by holding items of clothing (or whatever) close to her chest and either emotionally connecting with them or not. If she doesn't, it's out. She is also singularly strict about books and mementoes.

Warning: no menopausal woman should ever throw away mementoes. You are too fragile for a keepsake chuckout. Instead, what I'm suggesting is a small 'crap cull'. I tend to be a little more William Morris-esque than Marie Kondo in my approach here, working on the basis that, 'If it's neither lovely nor useful, but you can't quite bring yourself to bin it, then put it to one side and decide later'.

But what I'm trying to say in this chapter is that it's really tiring and boring being disorganized. So take a deep breath and do something about it. The house has been bunged up for years, it's screaming out for a good clear-out – think of it as giving the place a really good colonic irrigation.

Then, once you've done a basic sweep and actually delivered everything you want to get rid of to the charity shop (rather than leaving it in bags in the hall), you are ready to move on to Stage Two of getting your shit together . . .

. . . LIFE ADMIN

Buy some box files and label them – utility bills, car, health, bank, mortgage. Whatever needs filing, FFS file it. Dealing with your life admin efficiently will leave you more time to do the stuff you really enjoy. And knowing you have at least put your bills in a safe place will help you sleep well at night, whilst remembering to MOT your car will make you feel like the head of an important conglomerate. You are an adult – you can do this stuff; and once you start, it's like anything – yoga, walking – it will make you feel tons better.

CHECK-UPS

Remember, it's not just your car that needs MOTing. And the menopause isn't the only health issue most women in their fifties are going to face.

This is the time when you really need to start listening to your body. This is when the high blood pressure kicks in and when you need to attend all those scans and screenings, no matter how painful or embarrassing. No one likes getting their tits squashed between two metal plates, but it costs nothing and could save your life. So attend every check-up the NHS offers you. We are so lucky to have it – cherish it and use it.

Keep on top of your mail too. Don't ignore those reminders that come through the door from the optician and the dentist. Just make those appointments and go – you could be saving yourself a mountain of pain and heartache in the future. Your humble high-street optician could be the first to know you might be a glaucoma suspect – this happened to me in my mid-fifties and, ever since, I've been going for regular glaucoma check-ups, free of charge on the NHS at my nearest hospital. Yes, it's a tiny bit nerve wracking, but, as long as it's monitored and found early enough, glaucoma can be stopped in its tracks and some simple drops could prevent blindness.

EMERGENCY RATIONS

This is also the time to get ship shape. And I don't mean losing four stone and starting to run marathons. I mean by giving yourself more space to breathe.

There is something very therapeutic about clearing the decks. For starters, take control of your kitchen. Ask yourself whether a tin of kidney beans that went out of date in 2007 is really worth keeping (you don't even like kidney beans). And if a selection of discoloured lidless Tupperware containers land on your head every time you open a certain cupboard, bin them.

Next, make sure there are at least three proper meals you can instantly rustle up from store-cupboard items and yes, pasta and pesto do count. Restock your spice rack so that you can get a bit more creative with your basics and take a leaf out of Jamie's book by making sure you have all the staples required to make your weekly shop go further – stuff like red wine vinegar and miso, harissa spice and long-life cartons of white beans.

When everything else seems to be falling apart around your ears and you feel like your life is unravelling, taking control of your kitchen can feel like a big step towards feeling more on top of everything else. You might even get some weird kick out of re-arranging your cutlery drawer.

KIT YOURSELF OUT FOR ALL EVENTUALITIES

There is a special thrill that only a menopausal woman can experience when she knows exactly where something is. Life is so much easier when you have a special drawer containing stamps, ranging from emergency first-class, everyday second-class and pesky large, plus a large selection of envelopes, Sellotape . . . Oh God, I love stationery. I'm going to get really carried away here, Pritt stick – yes, glue, we all need glue – string, stapler, paper clips, wrapping paper and a great choice of postcards you can send to mates when they need cheering up/thanking/congratulating. Personally, I always package up my tax returns to my accountant with a card featuring David Bowie (I've got an assorted Bowie postcard box and I like to imagine one brightening up their office every quarter).

Oh – and a sewing kit. No one can afford to give up on a pair of trousers just because they're missing a button. Sewing on buttons can be really therapeutic, as long as you can manage to thread a needle without having a meltdown.

Finally, don't forget your first-aid box. Now you can really have some fun with this – hours in the chemist choosing your favourite antacids. And the one thing you don't need in this box is tampons. Any young menstruating visitor who comes on at your gaffe is going to have to shuffle down to the corner shop, knickers stuffed with loo roll, to buy her own supply, hahaha!

Sometimes it's great being older. As long as you're equipped to deal with it.

H

HORMONES

'The great thing about a hot flush is that you can defrost a tub of Ben & Jerry's in nanoseconds just by holding it against your big, fat sweaty neck. Hey presto – spoon soft!' **JE**

Ok, this isn't a science book. If you want to know what hormones are, I suggest you go on the Internet and do some research. However, unless you have a science degree, most of what you read will be pretty impenetrable. So in very simple terms (I've Googled this so you don't have to): hormones are chemical messengers in the body that travel in the blood to organs and tissues, signalling them to do the work they were designed to do. They can affect many different processes in the body, including reproduction, sexual function, metabolism, growth and development, and even mood.

A quick trip to your GP for a blood test will determine whether you are indeed menopausal or not. This test measures a hormone called FSH (follicle-stimulating hormone), levels of which are raised during the menopause, whilst other hormone levels drop.

Basically, we are all hostages to our hormones because they control our emotions, and when they start going haywire, we begin to malfunction. Imagine your body as a cartoon robot with a load of loose wires. Well, that's how the menopause can affect us. For many of us women, as soon as our oestrogen and progesterone levels drop, so does our ability to cope. But hormones don't just affect our feelings – they also have an impact on our physical wellbeing and there are many hormonal physical side effects that go hand in hand with 'the change'.

HOT FLUSHES

For some incredibly complicated scientific reason, diminishing levels of the hormone oestrogen can result in one of the commonest symptoms of the menopause: the 'hot flush' (or 'hot flash' as the Americans will wrongly insist on calling it).

The hot flush is one of the main reasons why women visit their doctor in middle age and the primary cause of lost scarves on buses. Most jokes about the menopause are of the 'Is-it-me-or-is-it-hot-in-here?' variety.

Middle-aged women who work in open offices are the ones I feel the most sympathy for. They're the ones, desperately trying to open windows, only for a half-dressed, shivering twenty-something to come along two minutes later and slam it shut. Life is far easier for those of us who work from home and can sit around writing books in our bras and pants.

For some women, the hot flush will be just that – a wave of warmth, similar to that you feel when you get off a plane in a Mediterranean climate – but for others it can be like stepping into Dante's Inferno, leaving the sufferer beetroot red with rivers of sweat running down her spine. Mother Nature can be very cruel when dishing out the hormones, which is why you will occasionally see women in their fifties divesting themselves of their coats in the supermarket and body surfing into the frozen-foods cabinet.

There are perks to the hot flush though. Central-heating bills can suddenly plummet and you no longer have any need for an electric blanket. But for many women they are an utter nightmare and the cause of much embarrassment. And the problem with getting embarrassed about something is that it can sometimes exacerbate the problem – in this case, the more self-conscious you feel about having a hot flush, the more dramatic its effects will be.

Society has come to terms with most bodily functions by now; television and the media have done a lot over the past few decades to shine a light on all sorts of health issues, and considering over half the population are female, hot flushes aren't exactly rare. But how many times have you seen a middle-aged woman hot-flushing in a soap? And why does no one ever pop in to see Doc Martin asking for an HRT prescription? The sooner women aren't made to feel like freaks for flushing, the easier it will be to deal with them.

Of course, the big question here is how hot is hot? When I went to the doctors about my own flushes and she asked this very question, I replied, 'Hotter than a burned-out Fiat Panda; hotter than a pitta bread that's just jumped out of the toaster; hotter than one of those patio heaters they put in pub gardens.' (Incidentally, these are very bad for the environment; in the future, they should scrap them and employ middle-aged women to waft around the pub garden instead, radiating more heat than the earth's core and keeping the customers toasty. They could pay us in Chardonnay tokens and everyone would be happy.)

Sadly, I don't rule the world. If I did, us lot would get the respect we deserve, and dry white wine would be freely available on the NHS.

HANDY HINT – HANDBAG FANS

Those tiny little battery-operated handbag fans can be very useful, so why not style it out and buy a selection to match all your outfits? Or why not customize yours, then pull it out at a business meeting like a sexy Bond weapon? Before you know it, everyone will be copying you.

Obviously, if you are the boss lady, then it's kind of your duty and prerogative to install a massive great fan in the boardroom – something that you can position strategically to make your hair stream out behind you like Rihanna in a pop video. (By the way, this look works best if you show a little bra – but only if it's a nice bra and not anything that looks a bit orthopaedic.)

HORMONES AND HAIR

There are many side effects to the menopause. On the physical side, the hot flush is the biggest problem for many women, but fluctuating hormones can play all sorts of other upsetting tricks on us girls and for lots of us it's either too much or too little hair in all the wrong places.

Many years ago, I was standing next to the actress extraordinaire Miriam Margolyes in the wings of a theatre. We were doing *The Vagina Monologues* (aptly enough) and one of the monologues was about a woman whose husband made her shave off her pubic hair which he considered dirty. With this monologue obviously in mind, Miriam whispered into my ear, 'I used to have such a luxurious bush before it all fell out.' I didn't know what she was talking about. I thought poor cow obviously had alopecia of the pudenda. But no, one of the facts of the menopause is that your pubic hair thins. What used to be thick and abundant starts to look very sorry for itself – all sparse and wispy and in my case a very drab-looking grey..

Of course what you 'lose on the chuff you gain on the chin'. Beards and tashes are the bane of the menopausal woman's life. This is when we start being unable to leave the house without a trusty pair of tweezers. Because for some women, by the time they've got off the bus and made it to the office, there's a fresh new crop ready for a ten-minute toilet break/pluck session.

The upside of all this growth is that there is little that is more satisfying than standing in a good light, with a really excellent pair of tweezers, tugging at a tough little bugger with a truly juicy root. Only people who practise the art of chin deforestation on a regular basis will know what I'm talking about here.

Joking aside, one of the most depressing hormone hair-related problems in middle age (or indeed at any age) is the thinning of hair on your head. We can all deal with a pubic area that looks like a neglected back yard, but losing one's crowning glory is a much harder pill to swallow.

For those of us who had lousy hair to begin with, the difference is harder to spot, but for some women FPHL (female-pattern hair loss) can be tricky to deal with. At this point, we have to remind ourselves it is not life threatening. Yes, it's tough but it will not kill you, and you will adapt. Find a hairdresser and a style that make the best of the situation, experiment with scarves and bandeaus and, if that doesn't work, don't suffer in silence: seek help. Remember, even when all this feels really shit, you are not alone. In fact, heat and hair loss are probably the two main symptoms that will prompt a woman to book an appointment with her doctor.

TO HRT OR NOT HRT?

There are all sorts of products on the market that promise to prevent you from suddenly boiling up like a turnip in a pan – some women swear by black cohosh, for example – but for many, hormone replacement therapy (HRT) is the only solution.

HRT replenishes the hormones you naturally lose due to the onset of the menopause. What you take and how is something to decide with either your GP or gynaecologist. There are many different brands and varieties, and although I've been happy on what I was initially prescribed, for some women it might be a case of trial and error.

Remember, your treatment can always be tweaked. Some people will feel happier on a plant-based type of HRT, whilst others might want to go down the bioidentical hormone route. Currently, there are over fifty different types of HRT on offer to menopausal women and, in my experience, there is almost certainly something out there that is going to help *you*. The type of HRT you will be offered will depend on a variety of factors, including the stage you've reached in the menopausal process and whether or not you've had a hysterectomy.

HRT might be taken orally in tablet form, transdermally (through the skin, via a patch or a rub-on gel) or as a slow-release implant. In some respects, it's like being back on the Pill again, and for some women this is not a path they want to take. In which case, there's a world of homeopathy on offer (see Chapter R for Remedies). I think every woman deserves to make her own informed choice and no one should be given a hard time for doing it 'their way'. Whatever gets you through the day, ladies.

However, HRT isn't suitable for all women and, as an alternative, cognitive behavioural therapy (whereby women are psychologically trained to deal with flushing episodes) has been proven more effective than you'd imagine. This is not to say that I belong to the 'it's-all-in-your-head' school of thought. I don't. But I do think that rather than fighting the flush and getting all hot and bothered about getting all hot and bothered, going with it might be a more practical way forward. I'd never be annoying enough to say 'embrace the hot flush', but I would say, unless you fancy medication, then your only choice is to accept it.

But let's not forget – it's not just women who occasionally sweat like dray horses pulling a cartload of barrels. Tony Blair, the former Labour Prime Minister, appears to suffer from hyperhidrosis (a condition characterized by abnormally increased sweating) and, if he once led the country whilst wearing sopping, sweat-soaked shirts, I think us women can let ourselves off the hook for getting a bit damp under the armpits now and then.

HRT AND ME

For me, taking HRT was a no-brainer, but I realize that now that sounds incredibly glib. Many women have medical backgrounds and family histories that rule it out, and for them it's medically not worth the risk. Others think it's cheating, but then there will always be a hard-core band of menopause hair shirts who are almost determined to make their experience as difficult as possible.

Some women genuinely don't feel they need it and that's totally cool, because let me say this until I'm blue in the face: every woman's menopause is entirely personal and we are all different.

I don't have a particularly low pain threshold. In fact, I think I'm quite tough. Show business teaches you to perform now and collapse later: I've been onstage with double-vision migraines, I once fell down an entire flight of stairs before I made my entrance and possibly did the whole show with concussion, and another time I threw up three times in the wings of the Theatre Royal, Newcastle when the norovirus hit halfway through a *Grumpy* show. I can normally soldier on – my dad was an army officer, for heaven's sake. I'm trained, I did a three-year course at drama school where I specialized in eating disorders and chronic jealousy. I can usually take any shit that's thrown at me and plod on.

But the menopause snuck up on me and felled me from behind. Obviously, I was kind of expecting it. I was over fifty and I'd been working on the *Grumpy Old Women Live* shows for a number of years. Together with Podcast Judith who is five years older and therefore well acquainted with her own hormonal weird-out, we'd written lots of middle-aged-female-related material, much of which centred around the peri-menopause and beyond. In fact, one of my favourite sketches (a brainwave of Judith's) in the first *Grumpy Live* show was called the Peri-menopausal Workout, performed with gritted teeth by Dillie Keane and set to increasingly frantic music. Essentially, it was a furious hormonal cardiovascular exercise routine that centred around domesticity rather than the gym, featuring Dillie demonstrating 'firming the waistline' by picking up all the mouldy mugs from under the beds, hauling sacks of potatoes home from the supermarket and ending with 'toning the upper arms' by slamming the kitchen cupboard doors. Dillie used to perform this routine with such rage it never failed to bring the house down. But for me, the peri-menopause was pretty non-existent – my tits didn't hurt, I wasn't particularly forgetful and I slept like a baby – which possibly lulled me into a false sense of security. I was going to be one of the lucky ones, I reckoned, so nothing had prepared me when, at the age of fifty-two, depression and anxiety hit me like a mudslide. I no longer felt capable of putting a cup of coffee down on the table without thinking it was in the wrong place. Every ounce of confidence seemed to drain out of the soles of my feet. I just wasn't 'me'.

Of course, it wasn't all doom and gloom. In amongst the depression and anxiety were sudden bursts of absolute uncontrollable rage. The kind that makes you a danger to yourself, the sort that makes you start shouting at the type of drivers who keep baseball bats in the boot – incandescent rage that had me spitting swear words in public, flying off the handle at the slightest provocation, swiftly followed inevitably by bursting into tears.

My family walked on eggshells. I was out of control. I went to see my GP.

I found him most unhelpful. So I saw a hormone specialist, got my HRT, went back to my GP and insisted he gave me in future what she had prescribed. Seven years later, I'm still on the same combination. I take Noriday (essentially the Pill) and rub two pumps of Oestrogel into my upper arm and, bingo, that's me sorted.

For me, the benefits of HRT kicked in pretty quickly and I remember the transition well. Because of my GP's reluctance to prescribe the stuff, I'd travelled to Australia to perform at a comedy festival with the stash my private hormone specialist had given me, but I hadn't started taking it. Did I really need it? Surely I wasn't 'that bad', I said. (My partner who had come out to Oz with me, looked dubious.) Then, the day after we arrived, finding myself weeping on the floor of my apartment in Melbourne, terrified at the prospect of performing my show, I decided to give it a whirl. Within a couple of days, I felt more like myself again, the show was up and running and my partner was no longer looking at me as if I might do something either stupid or dangerous or both. Ever since then, he has been HRT's biggest fan.

HORNY

One of the side effects of taking HRT is that it can reawaken a previously dormant libido.

I remember working with a particular actress who shan't be named (blonde, cockney), who used to come into rehearsals covered in carpet burns. When I pointed them out, she winked, licked her lips, thrust her hips and sniggered, 'Blame it on the HRT. I can't get enough – me and the old man were at it on the stairs this morning.'

Sadly for me (and the old man), this wasn't a side effect of HRT that I ever experienced.

1

INVISIBILITY

'Isn't it odd how a middle-aged woman who is twelve stone of solid fat and wearing a massive polka-dot frock can suddenly become invisible?' **JE**

So-called Invisibility Syndrome is one of the biggest bugbears of the menopausal brigade, ranking third behind hot flushes and forgetfulness. But, of course, the reality of this situation is that we're not invisible – we're just ignored.

For starters, try getting served in a busy bar when there is a constant stream of attractive young women vying for the barman's attention. Who is he likely to serve first? The twenty-four-year-old blonde in the crop top or the dumpy middle-aged blonde in that Boden shift that's seen better days? And who can blame him? Menopausal women are notorious ditherers and likely to change their minds three times before deciding on an order which they will then attempt to pay for with a twenty-euro note because they left their glasses in the ladies' toilets at work. Plus, the barman doesn't want to sleep with them. Therefore, they don't really exist on his radar.

As you get older, this happens more and more, and unless you are one of those women who hits fifty still turning heads, you will occasionally feel like someone cast a spell on you – because suddenly people seem to be looking straight through you.

Fact is, they can see you – you still physically exist – it's just that you do not merit any particular attention. You are not young, you are not hot, therefore what is your point? All everyone really wants is youth, and you, lady, are over the hill. Even the advertisers, unless they're selling nanna products, aren't really interested in you. One of the most shocking side effects of hitting the menopause, is that you and all the other women of a similar age get lumped into one big amorphous group labelled, 'beyond sell by'. This is when actresses find the work begins to dry up or that they're being offered 'granny-in-rocking-chair' roles. Meanwhile, in Hollywood, fifty-something men are being gifted on screen thirty-something girlfriends. This is because menopausal women aren't considered fuckable.

People stop paying attention to most of us in our mid-forties, when whatever cougar potential we ever had starts wearing off. Not that I had any in the first place. In fact, when I was younger, I used to joke about this – 'But I *am* foxy,' I'd insist. 'I'm foxy all right. I've got yellow teeth and I eat out of bins.' (I don't really. Well, actually, I do have yellow teeth, but I don't eat out of bins.)

As we approach fifty, people start looking straight through us because we aren't cute, we aren't sexy and most of us aren't rich. So what are we good for, really, apart from worming the dog?

Lots of women reading this will be shaking their heads in disbelief, including perhaps Madonna? (Who I don't believe has ever breathed a word about her menopausal experiences and instead would rather attempt to convince the world she has the ovaries of a nineteen-year-old and the dance moves to match.) But surely there has to be some common ground between Madonna and the rest of us. I do not want to deny my age, but neither do I want to spend the rest of my life being completely disregarded. My friend Podcast Judith says we should all take to the streets wearing high-vis jackets. But if I did that, someone would undoubtedly hand me a hard hat and shovel and expect me to dig up a road.

When Judith and I were writing *Grumpy Old Women: Fifty Shades of Beige*, we discussed invisibility and the following scenarios turned out to be our top three 'invisibility' bête noirs. Never mind no longer being wolf whistled at, these were the things that really got on our tits:

1. Waiters forgetting your meal, and then denying you ever ordered anything. Hold on, I'm a middle-aged woman – it's not very likely I'm going to go to a restaurant and not order any food, you fool.
2. Being left in the changing room in your bra and pants by an assistant who was meant to be getting you a bigger size and just forgot you were still there.
3. Being left at a motorway service station by your coach party (even though your partner got back on the coach but didn't notice you were missing because he sat next to another short-haired woman in glasses who might as well have been you).

Of course, there are steps you can take in order to make invisibility impossible. For some women, the menopause is a cue to introduce some eccentricity into their wardrobes. This is when some of us will hear the call of purple feathered hats and velvet cloaks, great big brooches and colourful tights, and my message to you is: go for it and fuck the dreary twats who laugh at you behind your back. Life is too short not to look however you like.

Life is also too short to lie about your age (unless I want a compliment, in which case I pretend I'm seventy-two, then sit back whilst everyone tells me how marvellous I look).

But being invisible isn't just about being overlooked physically, of nearly being run over on a zebra crossing because, 'Sorry love, I didn't see you!' (true story). It also goes hand in hand with being patronized.

On the whole, the world at large views middle-aged women as unimportant, and there is a communal glazing over when we speak. Which is weird, considering we are the ones who know stuff; we are the ones who could tell the supermarkets why their profits are down and advise the female fashion industry how to make their clothes fifty-something friendly (fewer synthetics, more width, more length, plus pockets and sleeves please). We might not be rich, but we often have control of the family purse strings, so ignore us at your peril. Remember, we are the customers who are deciding how your profits are going to look on a daily basis, because we're the ones looking at your shelves and choosing whether to buy or not. Don't underestimate us. Look around the supermarkets. Who is pushing the trolleys?

We're also the ones who pick the holiday destinations and which restaurant the family should celebrate a big birthday at; we are the ones who book the theatre tickets and day trips; we're the ones who drive the decisions to have a new kitchen, sofa, mattress, vacuum cleaner. People should be bending over to please us – it's not as if blokes are footing the bill on their own any more. And yet, most of the time, we're given the impression we're more trouble than we're worth.

Harrumph.

The weird thing is, not all middle-aged women are completely invisible. If you have money and are stepping out of your Bentley outside Claridges wearing that little Chloe number, then you will be completely visible. And the same is true if you are famous. Which I know because I once almost got mobbed at a motorway service station by a coachload of *Countdown* fans. I know it's not exactly Joan Collins territory, but you get the idea.

As a woman who is well known, but only in certain circles, it's really interesting to experience the difference between how I am treated by people who recognize me and those who don't. This will often depend on the demographic of where I happen to be. Say I'm staying in a hotel where there are a number of gay and/or middle-aged female bar staff, then the chances that someone knows 'who I am' go up. If the hotel is run by trendy young things, then – without exception – they won't have a clue. I should get the same treatment across the board, only that's not my experience.

What usually happens is, if I get recognized in reception, then I get a friendly smile and nice chat and possibly an upgrade. At this point, I will become utterly delightful – people are being nice to me, I'm nice to them, we are all having a lovely time in our bubble of niceness and because I am now in a good mood, I won't get all nit-picky about my room being too near a noisy lift and the fact that there is a used wet wipe in my bathroom bin – it's no big deal; the hotel might be a bit rough around the edges, but the staff are great and I would happily return. (Note: I have basically been shown the same courtesy that the average middle-aged man is shown as a matter of course.)

Consider the same scenario, however, when I am treated like Mrs Average. I will stand at reception for five minutes sighing loudly, whilst a young man or woman attends to something more urgent. When I do finally manage to get some attention, I will be referred to as pet or love, rather than Ms Eclair or Jenny, told my room won't be ready for another hour and no, they aren't taking any more lunch orders in the restaurant because it's gone 3pm (eye roll as if to say 'you imbecile'). Inevitably, when I do get to my room, I'm in such a foul mood I start looking for faults – the room is too near a noisy lift and there's a used wet wipe in my bin – and because the only way I'm going to get any attention around here is by complaining, I go into complete old-bag mode and start demanding to see the manager.

And the moral of this story is that if we were treated less like second-class citizens, we might stop behaving like first-class termagants.

For some women, becoming invisible in middle-age can be a relief, because it marks the end of getting a load of unnecessary attention. This is usually the case for women who, throughout their lives, have exuded more sex appeal than the rest of us. Surplus sex appeal has never been my problem. When #MeToo was gathering speed, I had to really rack my brains to think of occasions when I had been sexually harassed, and if I'm honest, I could count them on the fingers of one hand. But for my mate Julie who, from age fifteen to fifty could barely get on any mode of public transport without being ogled (bosoms, you see), sliding into sexual obscurity has come with a silver lining.

Without lashings of surgery, very few of us are going to be menopausal sex symbols. This doesn't mean to say we aren't fully functioning sexual beings in our own beds/up against the garage wall. But I honestly think that the more mature woman who cannot stop pouting in public starts to look a bit sad – though, at the risk of sounding bitchy, I guess if that's all you've ever had to offer, then it must be hard letting it go. But you know what? We all have to let go of something. Being sexy is great, being loved is even better, being admired is also very cool indeed and being respected is essential. Which is really what this chapter is all about.

J

JUMP AROUND

'My doctor told me I needed to do something cardio twice a week, something that got my heart racing and my blood pumping – so I took up shoplifting.' **JE**

Once upon a time, I was quite fit. In my thirties I used to swim most days and do yoga three times a week. If I'd only kept it up, by now I could be one of those flash gits in the fast lane at the local pool and yoga-wise, I'd be spinning on my head. But life got in the way, and heavens knows I'm lazy, so any excuse to break the pattern and I did.

Of course, my work doesn't help. The past few years have been very writing heavy and so – as a consequence – am I. Sitting in front of your computer for months on end can take its toll. I remember experiencing a sudden pain in my calf as I approached the end of my fifth novel, and being immediately convinced that I'd got deep vein thrombosis from not moving out of my chair. Typical, I thought. It's not as if I'm even flying long haul to somewhere exotic; I'm sat on my arse in Camberwell. As it turns out, it was just cramp and I lived to eat my tea.

At least when I'm gigging I burn a few showing-off calories. I'm quite a physical performer and I always come offstage in a sweat. But type as fast as you like, you're never going to really start perspiring;

there's nothing cardio about sitting in front of a computer all day. What's worse is that I write from home, so some days I daren't even look at my step app, because I know it's barely going to register double figures. All I do is walk from my study to the bathroom to the fridge and back. And I gave up smoking, which is great because it means my clothes don't stink of fags any more – but they don't fit either.

The healthier my lungs have got, the fatter and wobblier my thighs have become. I blame the old man, he's so good natured he's never once said, 'You've put on too much weight' – if only he'd nudged me when I first started piling on the timber. Honestly, it's all his fault. I blame Geof. Geof and the menopause, of course.

No one is quite sure if or why the menopause affects a woman's desire to move her butt, however a study into female rats who had their ovaries removed in order to mimic the human menopause found that they showed less activity on a running wheel over the next eleven weeks than those whose ovaries were still intact!

The evidence seems to indicate that a lack of oestrogen interferes with the dopamine receptors in the brain. As we all know, dopamine is the feelgood chemical and if that ain't there . . . well, we can draw our own conclusions. Only we can't because humans aren't genetically engineered rats. Hmmm – confused?

I have a friend from primary school who is six months older than me, but looks easily ten years younger, and I have a horrible suspicion that her secret is exercise. My friend literally jogged her way through the menopause. Somehow, as she ran around the park umpteen times, it seemed to fall away from her and never managed to catch her up. Consequently, she is still a size ten, her hair is thick and glossy and her skin glows. My friend is a primary-school teacher, she is practical and efficient, her life runs to a routine, she wakes up at the same time every day, eats a healthy breakfast and marches briskly to work, listening to a classic novel on her headphones. After a hard day of proper work (i.e. providing a future for other people's children and not mucking about on Twitter all day), my friend, headphones on, Dickens in her ears, marches briskly home. I'm not sure she actually had time for the menopause.

We all have a mate like this – one who looks at a hill and decides to walk it instead of catching a bus, even if it's raining and she's got an ingrowing toenail. We could all be a bit more like that efficient mate, who is still able to tuck a T-shirt into her trousers without a hint of a tummy bulge. But the fact is, for some of us, scheduling exercise into a non-existent routine is really hard, especially when one is out of shape and pathologically lazy.

Personally, I got a real wake-up call, mid-menopause when I eventually got around to going to the gym and a member of staff insisted on putting me through a series of exercises on weight-resistance machines. Unbeknownst to me, this circuit was specially designed to calculate my skeletal fitness in terms of age.

Well, the good news is that from the waist up I was a mere fifty-three-year-old girl. However, from the waist down I had all the strength of a seventy-five-year-old. Dear reader, I was fifty-eight at the time.

I'm not trying to play any blame games here. We all know how hard it is to fall in love with exercise when you've hated it all your life. The human race is roughly split on this one (just like everything else, it seems): some people are naturally inclined to go chasing after a ball, whilst the rest of us think, Sod the ball – look there's an ice-cream van parked just over there. However, the fact is that us menopausal women have things like bone density to worry about, so like it or not, we've got to keep moving.

BEFORE YOU START – KITTING YOURSELF OUT

This is the fun bit, where just by browsing in a sports shop you can almost convince yourself that you're already rather fit.

CLOTHING

Exercise clobber can be really expensive. There are all sorts of brands out there exploiting our insecurities, so if money is tight, a pair of jeggings and a T-shirt is as good as anything. I exercise in the same pull-up 'relaxed-fit' black trousers from M&S that I wear for just about everything – they're no trouble, they don't fall off, they're not too tight around the crotch and they wash like a dream. For me, the top half is the most important thing: you want it not so clingy that you cry when you catch sight of yourself in the mirror, but not so loose that it shows your tummy and bra should you be doing any bendy stuff.

Honestly, it was easier when we were at school and had a regulation gym kit that consisted of a brown pleated hockey skirt (the horror) and a yellow Airtex shirt.

UNDERWEAR

As with anything, the most important thing to get right is your foundations. You want a gripper knicker that doesn't slide around and a bra that keeps those puppies in place, especially if you decide to attempt jogging. There are loads of sports bras out there, some of them are even designed for 'high-impact' activities, which I think means they have built-in shock absorbers.

If you are big of knocker, then spending money on a good sports bra is vital, especially if you're serious about exercising regularly and don't want to go around looking like you're in an abusive relationship.

TRAINERS

When it comes to trainers, try and find some you like that aren't too cheap, but aren't going to bankrupt you either. I've got a pair of Adidas trainers which I bought seven years ago and still look brand new (which says more about how much exercise I do than the trainers, to be fair). But then I prefer my exercise barefoot and mat-based, rather than outdoor and boot campy.

WHAT KIND OF EXERCISE?

Now the one thing we can be grateful for is that there is a huge choice of stuff you can do to get your heart racing and your blood pumping, and I don't just mean looking at pictures of Keanu Reeves/Emma Thompson/the nice, fat butcher down the road (insert your own sex symbol here) – although masturbation, particularly if you do it really rigorously, must burn off a few calories, surely?

So, apart from energetic wanking, what else can you do to firm up and feel fitter? Well, basically, it's a matter of trial and error. Somewhere out there is a physical activity with your name on it and it might be . . .

PARK STUFF

Military-style fitness classes in the park. Now I'm slightly allergic to park boot camps. What I can't stand is the fact that they always seem to be led by some bloke in camouflage combat trousers who insists on screaming and yelling at the top of his voice, issuing billion-decibel orders, as if the motley bunch of Wednesday-morning, Dulwich Park school mums and hapless middle-aged women are being trained for some elite SAS swat team. Get over yourself, mate. That said, I know it works for some people and I've got a fifty-one-year-old journalist mate who looks forty from the neck down.

Parks are actually good places to get fit and quite a lot of them now have those machines that you can risk breaking your neck on. Make sure you are wearing suitable footwear (i.e. trainers) if you decide to have a go. Do not attempt any of this stuff if you are wearing those hessian wedges you bought for your cousin's wedding.

Your other park alternatives include walking around the thing. All the way around, mind you – not cutting through the middle, or even running around it. Loads of local parks hold Saturday morning fun runs, when you will be helped/encouraged to keep going by everyone else who is in the same boat. With any luck, you'll get swept along by all the enthusiasm. Alternatively, you can always pretend you've got a stitch, duck out and hide in the cafe.

RUNNING WITH AN APP

Running is anathema to me, but I do know people who were once as unwilling as me who have had a bash with that couch to 5K app and the results have been amazing.

The biggest problem with running (not that I'd know) is that some people (particularly some women) just aren't physically made for it. With big knockers, weak knees, flat feet and crappy ankles, they develop shin splints and jogger's nipple and occasionally throw up over someone's garden wall. Fact is, I would love to be able to run, to really give people a shock as I sprint with ease and elegance for the bus, but the reality is such a wheezing, bosom-holding, wooden-ankled stagger that people think I'm in the process of collapsing. So running just isn't for me.

SWIMMING

I believe that as long as you can actually swim, then being in water is one of the best things you can do to keep yourself sane. It's difficult to be depressed when the rest of your body is buoyant.

I used to be a really keen swimmer until I developed dry-eye syndrome (another menopausal treat – see page 233) which has made the whole experience much trickier, but it's still manageable as long as I wear goggles. And whenever I do go, I always feel so much better for it. Memo to self: go more often.

GYM STUFF

I joined a gym very late in life. I found one that offers scheduled classes as well as the usual circuit stuff. Booking is easy, it doesn't smell (yes, it does cost £60 a month, but for that price you can book as many classes and use the place as often as you like). Because I have a northern mean streak in me, I've worked out that as long as I go twice a week, I shall be getting my money's worth. This doesn't mean to say that I'm thrilled about my Monday morning cardio class, but apparently, it's going to get easier. Hmmm? The last time I finished the class, I was gym-shamed by a much older woman who told me, 'Don't give up, dear', as I exited the place looking like an advert for the dangers of hypertension.

CLASS STUFF

Exercise classes are great for menopausal women, they get you out of the house and are usually full of women just like you, only a bit thinner/fatter. These women could become your good friends, even if the only thing you have in common is a reluctance to get into your exercise gear and get moving.

Some exercise classes are very dance based, including zumba and anything else that involves your instructor having to yell above really loud music. These are my idea of hell. For starters, there is nothing worse than someone else's taste in music, plus I have no coordination – I cannot follow choreography to save my life. Not that my life's in danger; it's the woman standing next to me I'm more concerned about – the poor cow who is expecting me to jump to the right like everyone else and not to the left, a move which inevitably results in a visit to A&E to see if any of the delicate bones in her foot are broken. Whoops.

My favourite exercise classes are silent and mat based, with a relaxation bit at the end when you can start thinking about what you'd like for your tea.

I love a bit of yoga because I'm naturally quite bendy and it doesn't hurt as much as it looks like it should. However, I have no natural balance whatsoever and if ever we move on to tree poses, then I'm the one shouting 'timber' as I crash to the floor. My excuse for this complete lack of balance is the fact I have quite small feet in comparison to the rest of my bulk – I'm a size five and, really, if I'm expected to balance on one leg, then I could do with a pair of size nines. It's basic physics.

Even better than yoga is Pilates. Pilates is the ideal exercise for the bone-idle middle-aged woman. The great thing about Pilates is that it's a succession of tiny, controlled movements – so tiny, in fact, that no one can really tell if you're doing them or not! Consequently, if you drag your mat to the back of the class, you can lie down and have an hour-long kip by the radiators. Pilates is also the only exercise you can do immediately after a full English breakfast – another reason why it's so great.

CYCLING

Not everyone who is currently plodding their way through the menopause lives somewhere they can easily access a gym, fitness centre or church hall. Plus, some women hate the idea of memberships and communal classes. This is where cycling comes in.

Cycling is incredible if you like it. You can go anywhere for nothing and, after a while, you will start to develop that lean, sexy cycling body shape. That's if you don't get knocked off, of course.

Seriously, cycling is brilliant for so many people, but you have to know what you're doing, you must wear a helmet, have proper lights and preferably a high-vis jacket if you're out after dusk. Also, phone me when you get in, ok?

Even better than normal cycling is cheat cycling. The electric bike is the best practical joke any middle-aged woman can play on the cycling community. There is nothing like overtaking a much younger, fitter cyclist on a very steep hill, simply by triggering the ignition switch on an electric bike. I've borrowed one for a while in the name of research and life has never been easier. Electric bikes cost around a grand, which is pretty spendy, but just think of the cash you'd save on cabs. However, they're also quite chunky beasts and I realized if both me and the old man got one, we'd never be able to get in or out of our tiny little hallway.

HOME IN FRONT OF THE TELLY STUFF

For those who don't have access to a fitness centre and don't fancy cycling, don't think I'm going to let you off the hook – because as long as you've got wi-fi, you have no excuse. These days there are loads of online yoga and Pilates classes that you can do in the sanctuary of your own home.

Try *30 Days of Yoga* with Adriene, a lovely smiley Texan girl, who offers all sorts of yoga, from beginners to advanced in time slots to suit you. Even fifteen minutes of bending and stretching is better than nothing and you can fit a virtual class in to suit your schedule. Tougher and less loveable than Adriene is Cole Chance of YOGATX fame, but her classes, once you've got the basics, are really good.

If none of the above appeals, then may I suggest you get a group of like-minded menopausal witches together and play netball/rugby in a local pub car park. And if team sports don't appeal either, there's always the option of your own kitchen disco: dim the lights, put some music on and dance – really properly dance – for half an hour or at least until those oven chips are ready! Because literally any kind of exercise will give you a glow. And I'm not just talking about a big, red, sweaty glow. I'm talking the kind of glow that comes from within, thanks to the release of those feelgood endorphins that flood the body post exercise and temporarily mellow even the moodiest of us menopausal old bags. Try it. You might even like it.

K

KNITTING AND OTHER HOBBIES

'Who needs sex when you've got Twitter and knitting?' **JE**

When you were young, you didn't need hobbies. Hobbies were for sad people who had no mates to play with in the park – those weirdo kids who collected stamps and joined the Scrabble club. The rest of us were too busy snogging, smoking Embassy No 5 cigarettes and swigging cider to bother with boring old hobbies. But guess what? Come the menopause and suddenly hobbies are the way to go.

MY THING

The great thing about the menopause and realizing that you need something to take your mind off feeling like you may have gone a little bit bonkers is that you can rediscover things that you used to be quite good at but gave up when real life got in the way.

For me, hobbies are the mustards and pickles that add flavour to life. Finding one that is right for you might take time and patience – and remember, one woman's hobby is another's woman's massive yawn, so don't expect everyone to share your enthusiasm when you do find your 'thing'.

My thing happens to be drawing and painting.

Remember when you were little and were encouraged to draw and hours would go by with just a pad of paper and a few felt tips? Even as a child I found this therapeutic. As long as I was colouring in and drawing fashionable ladies in clothes I'd designed myself, I could forget about the trouble I was in at school and the page of maths homework with red biro crosses after every sum and a big angry '3/10, see me' scribbled across the bottom of the page.

Art was a safe world, and I was quite good, but sadly not good enough. By the time I was doing my art A-level it had become obvious that, whilst I had some flair, I never really had any talent. I watched the other girls in my group develop as proper painters – their figures were three-dimensional, they knew where the light came from and where the shadows went and they understood perspective as a matter of course. I was still just colouring in, really. I got grade D for my A-level, and I'm not blaming anyone, but after that I put my paints away for thirty-five years.

And this is a shame – because I missed out on thirty-five years of being able to calm my heart. Fact is, as I approach sixty, I'm still not very good, but I'm great at not being very good. What I lack in ability, I make up for in colour; I'm a very vulgar artist, I'm happy to say.

Because you know, one of the great things about getting older is that you don't mind being bad at something: I still don't get perspective, I still belong to what my brother calls the 'flat-earth' school of art. But I tell you, the ritual of taking all my art stuff from the cupboard and laying it out on the kitchen table, sharpened pencils, clean rubber, pristine paper, jewel-coloured paint pans is as soothing as a Japanese tea ceremony . . . and breathe.

The menopause can go on for around ten years, so you might as well spend some of that time learning things that will keep you company for the rest of your life.

ALL THE OTHER CRAFTY THINGS YOU CAN DO

People are often bewildered by the way middle-aged women suddenly get the urge to start doing things with wool. Now I've got a theory about this. I believe that once you stop secreting oestrogen, you start secreting another hormone and it's called the 'craft hormone'. This will manifest itself in various ways. For example, I found I suddenly got very turned on by the haberdashery department in John Lewis and the next thing I knew I was visiting hard-core crochet sites.

There is no point fighting the craft hormone – resistance is futile. And the great thing about crafting is there are so many different varieties to choose from, with lots of nice sitting-down hobbies for ladies who want to do something with their hands apart from opening the biscuit tin fifty times a day. Now, weirdly, there are women (my sister included) who fail to develop the craft hormone, and some go on to do an extra PhD instead. So apologies to those who find this chapter bewilderingly long and detailed, but for those who recognize themselves within these pages – fill yer boots.

KNITTING

Ok, for starters, wool is cheap (as long as you buy an acrylic mix rather than the fancy 100 per cent real-sheep stuff). Also, knitting needles are great. They're the only offensive weapon that you are legally allowed to carry on public transport. Personally, I am always tooled up when travelling.

Now there are many other things you can do with wool, but knitting is probably the easiest of all the wool-based activities, possibly because a lot of us learned the basics at school a million years ago. But the great thing about knitting these days is that the Internet is there to help you. If you need to remind yourself how to cast on (and off), then start by watching a couple of YouTube tutorials.

I've been knitting on and off for a number of years now and I'm probably ready to graduate beyond the simple thirty-two-stitch squares I've been making and sewing up for various dog/old people/charity blankets. And although occasionally I do surprise myself by using a few fancy stitches and patterns (Andalusian, Seed and the magnificent mitred square design), I still don't have the guts to go full-on 'garment'. (I keep encountering women on trains who are doing complicated things on three needles and wondering if they would mind if we used the journey as a private one-on-one tutorial. I'm quite happy to pay.)

Apparently, socks are pretty easy, but I'm not convinced, and the trouble with knitting patterns is that they're all written in Klingon. For example, what the devil does this mean:

K5, p2, k1, p2, k4. Rnd 4: K4, (p2, k3) x 2. Rnd 5: Cdd, k1, p2, k5, p2, k1. (12 sts) Rnd 6: K1, p2, k7, p2. Rnd 7: K2, p2, k5, p2, k1. Rnd 8: Cdd, k1, p2, k3, p2, k1. (10 sts) Rnd 9: K3, p2, k1, p2, k2. Rnd 10: K4, p3, k3. Rnd 11: Cdd, k3, p1, k3. (8 sts)

Hmmmm? No wonder women did all the code breaking at Bletchley Park.

Now, if like me you remain on the nursery slopes of knitting for the rest of your life and never move on to anything more complicated than colourful squares, don't beat yourself up. Charities are always looking out for blankets. All around the world people are living in the most dreadful conditions and I promise none of them could give a shit about the odd dropped stitch. Ok, so you can't knit a Fair Isle cardi, but you might be helping to keep someone warm at night.

Single knitted squares are also being used in premature baby units to introduce the mother's scent to a baby who is being incubated. Nothing is ever wasted.

Whatever your knitting ability, there is something very soothing about being in a wool store. The colours are so lovely and the shops are always run by nice people. And remember, if you can't knit, there's always . . .

. . . CROCHET

The world divides into those who can crochet and me. Try as I might, the rudiments of this yarn-based activity will not go in my head. I can make a simple chain, but as for turning that chain into anything more interesting than a series of random loops? Nope, it's not happening. I don't get it. Loads of people have tried to show me – in shops, on public transport – and I've spent hours in front of my computer screen, hook and wool in hand, only to have to leave the room and have a little cry because I just can't get the hang of it.

At this point, it might be best to admit defeat. We can't all do everything and even writing about bloody crochet is making me feel tense and I seem to be typing with a really clenched jaw, which is just ridiculous. But I mean kids can do it, and my mum's hairdresser makes these stunning blankets without breaking out into a sweat and there are all sorts of fantastic patterns and ideas out there and sometimes it just seems like there's a big old crochet party going on and I'm not invited and all I can do is press my nose up to this world of extreme crochet and bite down hard on my crochet hook whilst all the crochet people laugh. Sorry, but this inability to do something that by rights I should be able to do really hurts, and I'm going to have to leave the subject now before I disappear into a rabbit hole of 'crochet for idiots' YouTube videos.

And breathe.

(I was like this when I was a little girl too. I used to get so frustrated by not being able to play complicated skipping and ball games that I would take chunks out of rubber balls with my teeth and bite down hard on the wooden handles of my skipping rope. We don't change, we just get older.)

POM-POMS

Of course, for those who really are wool simpletons and can neither knit nor crochet, don't despair – there's a special pastime just for you. Yes, women, put down your needles before you do anyone a mischief, discard that crochet hook before you take your own eye out and welcome to the fabulous world of pom-pom making.

Ok, there are two ways of making pom-poms: the first is the method my mother would approve of – you cut your own pom-pom templates out of the back of a Cornflakes packet, like we did back in the 1970s; or, for the second, you go newfangled and purchase a professional pom-pom-making kit. These metal contraptions normally come two to a packet – one large, one small – and, once you've got the hang of them, will enable you to set up a pom-pom conveyor belt which will cause members of your family to exchange concerned looks behind your back.

The great thing about pom-poms is that they're 'in' right now, I made a couple of pom-pom garlands in neon colours last Christmas for gifts and the recipients pretended to like them, which is good enough for me. I also bought a pom-pom-making kit for an exam-stressed teenager and she got so instantly hooked, she stopped revising altogether – which, as you can imagine, thrilled her parents.

So a quick word of warning: pom-pomming is indeed one of the most addictive of crafts. Before you know it, you are buying speciality pom-pom-making books, which will lead you into a twilight world of pom-pom birds, fruit and animals – enjoy.

SEWING/STITCHING/EMBROIDERY

Sewing is harder than knitting because if you want to make something that is wearable, you need to use a machine. And a sewing machine is expensive, takes up a huge amount of space and you will need an engineering degree to understand how to thread the thing. That said, people I know who really can sew, make some pretty amazing stuff and save themselves a fortune.

I think I was slightly put off machine sewing by my mother's efforts to make clothes on the cheap for my sister and me. Back in the 1970s, there was something woefully unfashionable about homemade clothes. It basically meant your mum wouldn't take you to Miss Selfridge or Top Shop. Looking back, I was incredibly ungrateful. I remember being invited to one of my first mixed-sex parties (the birthday of a friend's older brother) in 1974, which was the year of the maxi skirt. I didn't have a maxi skirt (my older sister did, but I was far too fat to get into hers) and as the party approached, I became hysterical. Nothing else but a long maxi skirt, complete with a frill around the hem would do, and God bless my mother, she found a pattern, bought some floral-sprigged navy and white material and set to on the sewing machine. My mother only ever swore when she was sewing or knitting, but a good few 'God', 'damn', 'bugger' and 'blast it's later, a long skirt *with frill* had been produced. I wore it with a red puff-sleeved blouse and realized at the party that boys didn't really care what you were wearing. What they wanted was a girl with slight slag tendencies who would snog them in toilets. All that effort on my mum's part – completely wasted.

Sewing is like a martial art. It takes a really long time to get any good at it, but if you persevere you will end up like my friend Podcast Judith who can make curtains, which strikes me as one of the most grown-up things a woman can ever achieve. The rest of us will just spend the rest of our lives having flashbacks to sewing lessons at school where we spent an entire term bleeding over a wonky seamed apron.

TAPESTRY AND EMBROIDERY

A lot of what we call tapestry is actually embroidery, but let's not get too technical here. The great thing about both is that you can achieve quite remarkable results without too much skill.

Woollen tapestry kits are a big part of my hobby life. There are millions to choose from on the Internet. I go a bit mad and spend quite a lot of money on my kits, but when it comes to this type of thing, I do think you get what you pay for.

The trickiest kits are the ones that require you to follow a separate pattern, which basically means you have to concentrate like crazy and count stitches really accurately. The easiest – and the ones I insist on – have the pattern printed on to the background and are basically elaborate 'colouring-in-with-wool' jobs. The difference between colouring in with wool using a needle, and using a felt tip pen and paper, is that by the time you've finished it (give yourself anything from six months to twenty-seven years) you will have something of considerable beauty which you will want to keep. I get my tapestries turned into cushions via a charity called Fine Cell Work (@finecellwork) which aims to rehabilitate prisoners by teaching them sewing skills, be it quilt making or upholstering tapestries into cushions. Obviously, you pay for this service; it's around £50 per cushion, which may not sound cheap, but when you take into consideration the calibre of the craftsmanship and the fact that they supply all materials and the fabric is top-quality stuff (supplied by Osborne & Little, no less), it's completely worth it. Also, you are supporting people in pretty dire conditions to learn a new skill, earn a little bit of pin money and, with any luck, some self-respect. Of all the charities I've done business with, Fine Cell is the one I have seen make the biggest difference in people's lives.

PATCHWORK QUILTING

Quilting is yet another needle-based activity, which, if you get it right, can achieve some knockout results.

Older and Wider

My friend and fellow Grumpy Old Woman Lizzie Roper lost her much-adored father a couple of years ago. Pa Roper was a lifelong bon viveur and had a large collection of fancy silk ties. Painstakingly, Lizzie unpicked these ties and miraculously turned them into a large bedspread, which was then professionally quilted. The finished product is incredible and, although she has explained the process to me countless times, I still don't quite understand how she did it. Quilting is a time-consuming hobby and I think you have to have a great deal of patience, but it's ideal if, say, you've broken your leg or you're recovering from an op. For Lizzie, it was a way of taking her mind off her grief and making something that was both a memento and a homage to her dad – the centrepiece of the quilt is part of her father's Oxford University tie, complete with stain, proving, yet again, that things really don't have to be perfect to be beautiful.

I patchwork quilted a small cushion once when I was about seventeen and had (or was pretending to have) glandular fever. Looking back, I think I was in a stupor of boredom – basically, I wanted to leave school and the prospect of having to hurdle my A-levels before I could go to drama school did my head in, so I took a couple of months off, lolling on the sofa and generally opting out of revision. My mum gave me a great deal of help with that cushion. In fact, she finished it off for me, but I do remember it being really complicated.

Of course, these days, if you haven't got a mum around to help, there's always a YouTube video, and I know it's not the same, but at least the YouTube video doesn't tell you off.

OTHER CRAFTING HOBBIES
TO GET YOUR TEETH INTO

Of course not all hobbies revolve around wool and needles, the great thing about crafts is that once you've got bored of one hobby, there's another waiting to take its place.

PAPER CRAFT

Quilling. The utterly mindless and therefore totally satisfying Asian art of curling strands of paper and then manipulating them into shapes and patterns. Kits are available for under fifteen quid and will provide you with packets of rainbow-coloured strips of paper no more than a few millimetres wide which can either be hand curled or machine curled on a battery-operated tool (actually quite exciting). Templates are also provided for shaping your curled paper, plus glue and handy tweezer-type instruments for picking up your curled shapes and, before you know it, you're making really elaborate birthday cards which cost literally pennies but have taken you seven hours to create. Again, a quick Google search will very quickly introduce you to people for whom quilling is their life. There are some shit-hot quillers out there, mostly Japanese, who, let's be honest, are the champs of all paper art.

HIKARU DORODANGO

In fact, Japanese people are bonkers for all kinds of hobbies, and for those of you who have poo-pooed my ideas thus far, I give you *hikaru dorodango*. This is the ancient Asian art of shining dirt balls until they gleam like marble. The *dorodango* or dumpling is quite literally a ball made from mud and dirt, which is then painstakingly hand-polished over many hours until it is a smooth, gleaming sphere. Different soils will give different coloured balls and the results are really quite something. Fans of *hikaru dorodango* cite the meditative and healing qualities of time spent doing something which seems ridiculous but has spectacular end results.

Sorry to anyone who was bored rigid by this chapter. Not all of us can get our kicks in the same way, but for some of us (ok, me) various crafting hobbies have helped keep me (relatively) sane during the menopause and, as a result, even my thirty-year-old daughter has taken to keeping a 'stress ball' of knitting handy for when she needs to stop fretting and properly wind down.

PS Recently, Podcast Judith and I went on a residential two-day 'beading' course at Denman College, which is the HQ of the Women's Institute in Oxfordshire. Here, we spent an incredibly happy time making ridiculously intricate Christmas decorations. I know some women would rather spend their money on a spa break but being pampered has never really done it for me, so this all-inclusive 'craft jolly' was my idea of pure indulgence. BTW, you don't have to be a member of the WI to attend Denman, though there are hefty discounts if you are.

L

LIVE, LOVE, LAUGH!

'I recently stayed in a farmhouse in the Lake District which had a visitors' book. All the other guests had written pleasant things, like, "Super property", "We'll be back", "Loved the Aga and the cheeky little robin in the garden". I wrote, "Porn shoot went well".' **JE**

Listen, I'm not entirely taking the mick, but the title of this chapter is very much tongue in cheek – because the world divides into those who like hand-painted signs telling them how to go about their business and those who would like to burn the fuckers! And guess which side I'm on? Hint: I'm the woman with the kerosene and the matches.

But putting raging cynicism to one side for a moment, choosing how you want to live through the menopause is very much your decision to make. You can go through the process biting off everyone's heads and then sobbing in the toilets, or you can come clean and tell everyone you're struggling and that you need a bit of help. In fact, rather than all these 'Live, love, laugh' items that are so readily available, maybe we need someone to design us a T-shirt emblazoned with the words: 'DEAD INSIDE'.

Ahem, and this is me putting my cynicism to one side!

Of course, as with everything, we need to find some middle ground here. No one is expecting you to go through a massive hormonal upheaval like some kind of middle-aged Pollyanna, finding the silver linings in even the most gruesome of side effects: 'Insomnia – yay!' But the alternative, which is to be permanently livid and resentful for the duration, is equally unattractive.

We only get one go at life, and considering the menopause can drag on for a decade of your allotted time on this planet (plus an extra couple of years for the peri-menopause) it would be a shame to waste that time by being permanently down. So, with that in mind, let's put a positive spin on the menopause – the most important things to remember are:

1. It's not going to kill you. The menopause can be upsetting and inconvenient, but it's not going to put you in a hospital ward for months on end. There is nothing about the menopause that should cause any real chronic physical pain, so if that's what you're feeling, get down to your doctors ASAP; don't blame every ache and health niggle on the menopause – there might be other stuff going on, so get it seen to.

2. It's not going to last for ever. In fact, if you decide to take medication, you may barely even notice it's happening. Some days will be easier than others, but there is nothing about the menopause that should leave you with any long-term damage. Possibly the biggest hormone-related worry is osteoporosis (brittle-bone disease, leading to fractures) and any woman who has a history of this condition in the family should take all the precautions she can to prevent it.

3. You are still young. Old age is far more fraught with danger than our middle years. As my mother says, 'Being ninety isn't for cissies'. But let's get through this bit first!

What we all want is to live well through the menopause, not to fall out with the people we love and have as much fun as we can cope with, but still be in bed by 11pm. (Who am I trying to kid? Most nights I'm up those stairs on the dot of ten.)

To be honest, I have quite a low threshold for 'fun', but I do like to enjoy myself. It's just I enjoy myself differently these days.

The other evening our young neighbours had a party that spilled out into the garden and eventually wound up at around 8am. It was approaching 9am by the time the last bodies had crawled indoors. Meanwhile, next door, I was up and dressed and coming downstairs for breakfast, and as time passed, I could feel how shit they were feeling through the walls – their hangovers were almost forming damp patches and no one on their side of the wall stirred for the entire day. I, on the other hand, did some yoga, a line of tapestry (the new cocaine), smashed a boiled egg on to some avo toast and went out to see the Van Gogh exhibition at the Tate Britain. Now that's what I call having a good time.

One of the most interesting revelations about the menopause is that, for many of us women, it's a time of discovering who we really are, what we really like and what we really can't be bothered with. By the time you are menopausal, a lot of life stuff may have already slotted into place. If you're going to have babies and a career, then you will probably have already gone down that road, although, as we all know, careers are something you can change at any time of life. But what I'm trying to say is that for the majority of women, by the time we stop ovulating we will have reached a stage in our lives when we more or less know who we are.

As a younger woman I spent so much time competing and trying to be a more exciting version of myself that I often lost sight of who I was. One of the perks of the menopause is that you finally come to terms with the kind of woman you are, and if there's anything you don't like about yourself, then you'd better deal with it pronto.

Or don't. It can only be up to you.

For me, I've entered the 'like-it-or-lump-it' time of life, meaning that if I don't like something, then I either change it or I put up with it, but I refuse to obsess about it any more. Yes, I'm infuriated by my dumpy cellulite-riddled legs, but if I'm on a beach and I fancy a swim, then the sarong is coming off. Life is too short to miss out on a nice swim in the sea. Because I've realized – no one is all that interested; I am not the dumpy-legged star attraction of the beach. (Although, indubitably, further down the beach there is probably another very similarly sized woman nudging her mate and saying, 'Her, then? Am I dumpier than her?')

Everyone has something they hate about themselves, but if you haven't come to terms with whatever this is by the time you're menopausal, then you are in danger of becoming rather boring and shallow. Your friends don't love you because you're perfect; they love you because maybe you're quite interesting, you listen, you're loyal and you can have a laugh.

And that's the great thing about being older. We can be who and what we choose to be. We can be the us we've been wanting to be for years, or as David Bowie once said, 'Ageing is an extraordinary process whereby you become the person you always should have been.'

So the menopause is a great time to start being honest with yourself and the people around you. This is when, deep down, you finally know your own mind. You know which flowers you really like and that even buying a small bunch of them will make you feel like a queen; you know whose company you enjoy and whom you are best avoiding. This is the silver lining of the menopause – a wealth of experience to help you through the crappy bits. You are old enough to know who your favourite authors are and what kind of books you like to read, you don't have to try Campari and soda to know that it's hideous and that you much prefer a nice chilled Chardonnay, you've been around the block, you know by now if you're allergic to shellfish. You can relax; you've made most of the mistakes you are ever going to make.

There is huge comfort in knowing so much about yourself. You know what will make you miserable and what will brighten you up. Small things that cheer you up are like stepping stones through a muddy stream, so if you're having a crappy day, try and remember what those stepping stones are. Mine include fifteen minutes of yoga on my mat, a cup of coffee made with hot milk, and a bath. You have to know how to comfort yourself – your mum is too old now. Here's some other stuff I use:

- Big, fat family sagas on Audible. I find Audible incredibly comforting when I'm anxious. I like Penny Vincenzi or Julian Fellowes or, for the ultimate in comfort reading, *The Cazalets* by Elizabeth Jane Howard.
- Food is another thing that makes us feel either great or foul. Try not to choose the stuff that is only going to make you feel awful ten minutes after guzzling – my go-to cheer-up nibbles are fruit and cheese and sometimes I pick all the nuts out of a box of nutty muesli.
- Cheer-up telly. It's great to have a box set up your sleeve for when the world has gone slate grey. I love *Brooklyn Nine-Nine*, any old Alan Partridges and the entire *Peep Show* back catalogue.
- Have a hobby that you can pick up easily, so you don't have any excuse not to do it. For my birthday last year, Podcast Judith

bought me a knitting bag – once upon a time I'd have put it over her head, now it goes everywhere with me.

- Be kind to yourself. And try to be nice to other people – if you have been a cow, apologize. Tell your family you love them and you're sorry if you've been difficult; tell them what's going on and try to have a laugh about it.

Laughing is so important. We are told all the time about how vital it is to eat healthily and exercise our way through the menopause, but now and again we need to be reminded that it is equally as important to laugh. Laughing is so liberating. It takes us back to being children; it's a pure, uninhibited response and we need to do it as often as we can. I have mates who are guaranteed to make me laugh on the phone. Even when they are telling me woeful tales of terrible things, they will still make me laugh. In fact, I once laughed so hard at one of my friends I shat my pyjamas. I have been chasing that kind of laugh ever since.

My mother makes me laugh and my daughter makes me laugh. My daughter makes me laugh with a kind of shorthand only the two of us share. I like laughing at her and the sound of her laughing at me is one that gladdens my heart.

My partner makes me laugh too, quite often when he doesn't mean to. He makes me laugh when he gets completely furious about something and starts swearing under his breath and he makes me laugh when I see how happy he is to have an ice cream and he makes me laugh when I ask him to boil me an egg and when I take it out of the pan I find that he has drawn a face on it. (He has been drawing faces on my eggs ever since we got together thirty-seven years ago. Who needs to ovulate, when you have hand-drawn faces on your hard-boiled eggs?)

M

MOOD SWINGS

'*Don't talk to me about mood swings. I'm a one-woman mood-swinging metronome. I can swing from miserable cow to hysterical bitch in a nanosecond.*' **JE**

The worst thing about mood swings is feeling like you've lost control. If like me, you struggle with your emotions, regardless of any hormonal imbalance, then this can lead to making a fool of yourself on a regular basis – arguing on the street, causing silly Twitter storms, bursting into tears on public transport and kicking inanimate objects which inevitably leads to breaking your own toe.

I think a good outburst is worth its weight. I like to have a bit of a scream, bite down on a wooden spoon and then do swearing – really foul-mouthed 'fuck and cunt' swearing – until, like a giant toddler I tire myself out. Other women eat chocolate, which is fine, as long as you don't end up in a vicious cycle of self-loathing. I'm not a chocolate lover, but I have been known to hit the Chardonnay, which we all know is silly, because you are going to have to go through the same old shit the following day, only then it's going to be a billion times worse because you've got a hangover.

If we could be rational, then we know what we should do: some deep breathing, or even ten minutes of yoga. Hell, even ten minutes of colouring in is better than going on a neighbourhood rampage because someone didn't scoop their dog poop from outside your front door.

But how do we keep the lid on the pressure cooker of our tempers? Because tantrumming at our age is so not a good look (unless we do it behind closed doors, in which case I reckon it's really cathartic).

TRICKS FOR KEEPING YOUR COOL

- Make sure you're not literally overheating – always give yourself the option of being able to remove items of clothing that are making matters worse. Avoid polo necks.
- Sniff some lavender; keep some essential oil handy at all times and rub it on your wrists. At least then if you do lose it, you'll look terrible but smell great.
- Count to twenty. Ten is never enough.

What we all need is to be kind to ourselves without being self-indulgent. If and when you have behaved badly, apologize and mean it, and then allow yourself a treat for being such a big girl.

Treats come in all shapes and sizes, for me it's cheese and a handful of crisps, time out with a good book and maybe a couple of rows of therapeutic knitting, followed by a quick browse through the David Austin rose catalogue (no one can be angry when they're looking at roses).

Swimming, walking, talking to a mate, painting your toenails – there are a million ways to cheer yourself up. The trick is not to be so fucked up you won't even help yourself.

A word of warning here, menopausal mood swings come in many different guises, and I for one am quite capable of running through an entire catalogue of different emotions in a single day, usually involving tears followed by laughter, creating a sort of daily menopausal rainbow of moods.

FURY

Anger doesn't often appear on the list of 'common menopausal symptoms' but for me it was one of the hardest things to control.

It was also one of the most dangerous. I live in south-east London where it's not advisable for dumpy middle-aged women to start shooting their mouths off, but God help the cab driver who stops his black cab to offload litter on to my street, only to find that I am picking it up and shoving it right back through his window. (After a brief exchange of insults, he realized what he was dealing with and drove off, but I gave chase, taking down his registration number and yelling abuse. As he sped off around the corner, I caught sight of his face in the wing mirror. He looked terrified.)

As the menopause kicked in, I became incredibly confrontational, constantly itching for a fight. I could barely drive for half a mile without getting involved in some kind of road rage. The inside of my windscreen needed saliva wipers as I spent so much time hissing and spitting, my knuckles white from frenziedly gripping the steering wheel.

Rude gestures and tooting weren't enough. Most incidents called for full-blown slanging matches which included stopping the car, getting out and screaming in the middle of the road – usually at some poor sap who had accidentally cut me up at the lights and was now being subjected to a verbal battering.

I have always been a slightly bad-tempered woman, but this was full-on Jekyll and Heidi stuff. I felt murderous and violent. I wanted to break things and lash out, I wanted to push teenagers off their bicycles for pedalling on the pavement and throw unscooped dog poop at pet owners' heads. My jaw was almost permanently clenched and I needed new swear words because I'd worn out all the ones I knew.

The problem was (as my eminently more sensible partner pointed out) that, with this kind of behaviour, I was in danger of getting punched in the face, or worse. He was genuinely scared that I was capable of getting mixed up in something really dangerous and didn't like me going out unaccompanied.

Looking back now, I should have channelled all this furious energy into something that would have done me good, like kick boxing. But I was too angry to use my temper to any positive effect and eventually the only time I wasn't angry was when I ran out of temper and felt exhausted, weirdly vulnerable and scared of just about everything.

ANXIETY – THE FLIP SIDE TO ANGER

Of course, the flip side to anger is snivelling fear and anxiety, and when I wasn't stomping around, pushing kids off bikes and shoving burger wrappers back into black cabs, I was indoors, wishing I could stay under the duvet with the curtains closed.

This wasn't all day every day. In fact, a lot of the time, I'd wake up feeling quite normal. But then I'd be gripped by these unexpected waves of utter desolation when everything seemed utterly hopeless and pointless, and for twenty minutes or so I'd be convinced that I was the biggest waste of space on the planet. I'd be gripped by sudden irrational fears, my hypochondria (which has always been pretty awful) would go into overdrive and there wasn't a week that went by without me imagining some dreadful disease.

Looking back, I feel quite cross with myself. Your fifties are often a fraught time, and whilst I knew people who were genuinely struggling with tricky diagnoses, there was me, making up catastrophes in my head. But nothing is logical to someone who is grappling with anxiety, and I spent a good while convinced that if *I* wasn't dying, then something terrible was going to happen to a loved one.

The worst thing about this type of fear is that it sometimes comes true. My dad did die; he was ninety, he was old and tired of being ill and the reality of his death was somehow easier to deal with than the fear of it. Which doesn't mean to say I don't miss him. It's just that my memories of him are so vivid that it's very easy to imagine he's still here, and I know it's mad, but sometimes I think that if I walked into my kitchen to see my father sitting there, I wouldn't be the slightest bit surprised. Mind you, I still think I might bump into my nanna, which is pretty impossible considering she'd now be 120 and is long dead.

Anxiety can strike at any time. My daughter, who was between flat-shares at this time, was living at home and consequently my nerves were on constant vibrate. She was in her twenties and yet if she was later than expected after having her hair bleached half a mile down the road, I'd be convinced she'd been abducted. I lost all sense of proportion. I hated her going out and I'd wake up in the middle of the night, desperate to know if she was safely home. If she wasn't, I'd take up position in the old man's study at the front of the house, pull up the roller blind and wait for the night buses to roll up the hill. The glorious thing about living opposite a night-bus stop is that I could physically watch her get off the bus, cross the road and then hear her put her key in the door. At this point, I would run back to my own bed and pretend to be a normal sleeping human being. Yet the truth is that sometimes I was in such anguish I would punch myself in the head.

WEEPINESS

I'd say I'm an average crier. I'm not one of those women who sobs at every little thing, but on the other hand, *Call the Midwife* gets me every time. Fact is, the menopause turned me into more of a weeper – mostly tears of frustration at buttons falling off coats, lost car keys, really looking forward to smashed avo on toast for breakfast only to cut into said avo and find it had gone all mushy and brown inside. Boo-hoo-gnash.

I also became incredibly sentimental. Telly ads would have me welling up, little girls holding their mother's hands in the super-market would trigger a huge lump in my throat and once, driving past my daughter's old school, I had to pull over whilst I wept for twenty minutes – great, heaving, wracking sobs of nostalgia for a life that I'd once had that was now over.

Now the biggest problem I have with crying is that it makes me look very ugly. Some women can cry quite prettily; these tend to be oily-skinned brunettes – the great thing about oily skin is that the tears just roll off it. However, those of us with rubbish pale and dry skin are kind of allergic to crying – we blotch up dramatically and look like we've got a terrible case of measles within ten minutes. Plus, my face tends to swell up and it's not an attractive sight.

LETHARGY

Having spent many years working from home, I've always given in to the temptation of an afternoon kip, sloping off at about 4pm for a quick half hour, two or three times a week. But when the menopause hit, I started craving my bed even as I was making it first thing in the morning. It would be 9am and I'd be wishing it was late afternoon so that I'd have an excuse to crawl back under the covers. The days seemed to go on for ever, my legs felt like sand bags, my brain felt like it was going in slow motion, even typing felt like hard work, whilst the idea of going out for dinner or to the theatre filled me with dread. The prospect of leaving the house was exhausting. Could I really be bothered?

The only time I felt my pulse really beating was when I was onstage. Dr Theatre is an incredible thing and, however angry, tired, anxious or down I was, performing never failed to pick me right up. Being onstage can be a bit of a refuge from the rest of the world: for a few hours you cannot think of anything else – you have just one responsibility and that's to entertain your audience. Sometimes things are easier when they're kept simple – if you've got the one job, you can do it and gigging was always my safe space.

JEALOUSY

That said, as I progressed through my very menopausal fifties I was aware that work might not continue to fall into my lap as it had in my forties. Realizing your career is stalling can feel like the last menopausal straw for a lot of women and, sadly, statistics prove that whilst men of, ahem, mature years will continue to be promoted right up until retirement, women are often sidelined and end up staying put.

Now I have very little experience in the world of real work, but for me in my ridiculous showbiz/writer's bubble, I could feel a shift in the type of work I was being offered. Basically, the telly stuff dwindled – not that I'd ever been hot telly property – but after the third-place success of *I'm a Celebrity* in 2010, which led to a year's stint on *Loose Women*, the big opportunities got smaller. By the time I was fifty-five, I had to come to the conclusion that, TV-wise, I'd peaked and from now on I'd be lucky to get offered the odd one-off appearance.

Let's be honest here. I did feel shit about this. And I was jealous. I was jealous of all the new funny, younger women who were being discovered and promoted above my head. Watching those who had been chosen for telly jobs I would have killed for did my head in, my already fragile ego shattering on a nightly basis. For me, the answer was simple. I started turning the box off . . .

And breathe.

Netflix has been an absolute gift for a jealous old bag like me. I can settle down in front of a nice black and white movie rather than sit seething in front of panel games that have chosen to overlook my talents.

I'm lucky; my demons can at least be controlled by pressing the Off button on the remote control. I imagine it's a lot harder for many other women in proper jobs up and down the country. Feeling like you're being passed over can be difficult to deal with. It can also make you bitter and nasty, which will add to the reasons why people don't want to employ you. So you've got to watch that. In my experience, it's best to keep bitterness under your hat. Don't let it slip out in public – it won't do you any good.

Eventually, you will learn to process your jealousy or use it to your own advantage. In my case, feeling like I'd been scrap-heaped made me even more determined to keep proving myself and I started working harder, ultimately producing the most successful touring show of my career. *How To Be A Middle Aged Woman (Without Going Insane)* carried me through my mid- to late fifties. I also stopped fighting the natural direction my career had begun to take and now I don't really think about the jobs I don't get and try to concentrate on the stuff I *have* got instead – the books and magazine columns and, of course, the *Older and Wider* podcast.

As such, I have become the mistress of my destiny. My success or failure is kind of up to me; it's certainly not up to some telly executive (although that said, if any one of those telly execs fancied offering me a nice sit-down afternoon quiz show, I would quite literally bite their hand off).

SOLUTIONS TO THE MOOD SWINGS

For me, the mood swings at the beginning of my menopause were much harder to handle than the physical symptoms, and there were days when I thought I was losing it completely. In the end, when neither myself nor the old man could stand it any longer, I marched myself down to the doctor's – because sometimes you've got to hand yourself over to the experts. I was offered HRT, which helped not only my menopausal physical symptoms, but also my temper. My partner noticed the change within days.

Sometimes women are offered antidepressants rather than HRT. This is something you have to weigh up and decide whether to go for them or not. Personally, I'm grateful I've been able to take a medication that dealt with the root of the problem, which was definitely hormonal, rather than 'in my head'. I'm not against antidepressants, but I'm not sure I agree with using them to deal with menopausal symptoms.

TIPS

1. Experiment with different types of exercise to alleviate different symptoms. If you're feeling angry, sign yourself up to a box-ercise class, personally I find yoga great for days when I feel really stressy.

2. Choose something nice to wear. Don't self-sabotage – don't make matters worse by wearing the itchy jumper and the uncomfortable trousers.

3. Have a bath. Some women swear by magnesium baths to ease anxiety. Magnesium is a mineral that helps the nervous system to relax, so a nice hot Epsom salts bath, particularly for those who carry their tension in their muscles, can really help at the end of a tough day.

N

NIGHT SWEATS AND INSOMNIA

'*The trouble with overheating in bed and ripping off your nightie is that your partner thinks it's a sexy come-on and starts getting excited.*' JE

Night-time is the worst time for anything, isn't it? All around the world, whenever it's dark and we're all meant to be tucked up and sound asleep, millions of menopausal women are turning over their pillows, kicking off duvets, traipsing to the toilet for the umpteenth wee and trying not to panic about the sheer amount of moisture that is seeping from their bodies. Friends of mine say, at times they have felt like human sponges. In fact, I once met a woman who told me that when she was at her menopausal worst, sweat would literally drip off her nipples.

Night sweats are a common symptom of our old friend 'plummeting oestrogen levels'. For some reason, this drop causes the part of the brain that acts as the body's thermostat (the hypothalamus) to malfunction, thinking the body is overheating. This, in turn, triggers the body's usual attempts to keep cool i.e. the skin reddens and the sweat glands start working overtime, which for some sufferers means changing the sheets at silly o'clock or sleeping on top of towels.

Anything that interrupts your sleep is a bore because, after a while, it affects your ability to function the following day and you will find yourself nodding off at your desk, just like you did when you were at school and couldn't stay awake during physics. Even if night sweats are part and parcel of a bog-standard menopause, the consequences can be dramatic. Accidents happen when you're tired and it can be dangerous to drive long distances when you've been awake since dawn. Tiredness can affect every aspect of your life, making you clumsy and forgetful – this is when you end up in A&E for simply preparing vegetables and being too knackered to be careful; this is when you will suddenly forget your PIN, even though you knew what it was twenty minutes ago; this is when you will pretend to need the loo at work, just so you can sit down for five minutes; and this is when you fall asleep on the 176 bus, miss your stop and end up in Penge.

Tiredness is one of the most debilitating side effects of the menopause, although it's important not to blame everything on the change in your hormone levels. So if you are constantly knackered, pop in to see your GP – your thyroid could be playing up and a simple blood test can check if everything is functioning properly.

Of course, if you share a bed with someone, not being able to kip can be made worse by feeling guilty about disturbing your partner's beauty sleep, hmmm? There's always the option of the spare room or the sofa . . . for them, not you! You're already having a miserable enough time without having to go and lie on the lumpy old spare-room mattress or the sofa that smells of old curry stains.

Most people are a liability in a shared double bed. If one of you isn't sweating like a dray horse, then the other is snoring like a hedge strimmer. But then again, when my partner isn't being a nuisance at night and is just lying there perfectly still, not making a sound – not even that awful whistling-down-his-nose noise – then I panic and I think he might have died. We can't win.

For some women the interruption of a normal sleep pattern can set in and it can be very hard to shake off. This is when the bogeyman insomnia can move into your bedroom – and insomnia can be a pig to get rid of.

As a woman who could normally kip on a washing line, the menopause was a very rude introduction to suddenly not sleeping through the night. For me, it was mostly needing a wee that had me padding from my bed to my bathroom, but once I was awake, hormonal anxiety could have me quaking under my duvet for a couple of hours on the wrong side of midnight. So, although my insomnia wasn't night-sweat induced, I do know what it's like to lie awake in bed, counting down the hours until dawn, and it's not something I would wish on anyone.

My brush with what I would call proper insomnia happened when I accidentally brought bed bugs back to my London bed from a posh hotel in Norway. I'd done the classic thing that all travel websites warn you not to do: I put my case on the bed to pack for our return flight and a couple of the blighters obviously hitched a ride home with me. Once they were safely installed back at my place, they started to breed, and within weeks a few had probably turned into a few thousand (that's the nature of bed bugs). It took me six weeks and a grand's worth of fumigation to get rid of them, and because I was so traumatized by these events, it took several months before I could relax sufficiently to get a decent night's sleep. I became paranoid, convinced I could feel them, hear them in the wooden framework of my bed. I used to hate bedtime.

Throughout this bout of poor sleeping, I felt like a basket case on a daily basis, so I have every sympathy for anyone who is losing precious zzzz through night sweats, because once your sleep pattern is upset, it's very difficult to imagine you will ever sleep properly again.

Believe me, you will, but it may take some time.

Having talked to friends about night sweats, the same kind of scenario that I had with the bed bugs arises, you go to bed dreading what might happen and inevitably the fear of the night sweat becomes as bad as the night sweat itself. Anxiety breeds anxiety and night-times can be the very worst for lying there fretting about everything, with each nagging doubt weirdly magnified by the dark. How many of us have lain awake worrying about something which seems like a massive worry at four o'clock in the morning, only for the problem to shrink into something quite trivial as soon as day breaks.

I think the only way to approach a dodgy menopausal sleep pattern is as practically as you can.

TIPS FOR GETTING A BETTER NIGHT'S SLEEP

1. Make sure your bed is as comfortable as possible; start by giving it a good airing and brushing out all the old toast crumbs.

2. Ensure your curtains or blinds block out the light sufficiently. If not, you can experiment with sleep masks and pretend you are flying first class to Barbados every night.

3. A new mattress might be extortionately expensive but a new mattress topper is a great deal cheaper and can make all the difference.

4. I've found that, although I wouldn't dream of ironing sheets,

ironing pillowcases makes the bed feel infinitely more luxurious and a teeny bit like you might be staying in a posh hotel.

5. Try popping a chocolate on top of your pillow for that extra
four-star touch. Though make sure it's wrapped. I once accidentally kicked a pillow chocolate down the bed where it
melted all over the bottom sheet. In the morning I woke up
to find what looked like poo all over the bedclothes.

6. Make sure your bedroom is as calm as possible. Even if the
rest of the house looks like Steptoe's yard, try and make your
bedroom the one place where you're not tripping over yester-
day's knickers.

7. Always make your bed when you get out of it in the morning.
Even if you just want to crawl back into it, straighten it up
– because there is nothing more likely to guarantee a poor
night's kip than climbing into a pile of tangled limp sheets at
the end of the day.

8. Declutter the space immediately around your bed. Make sure
your bedside table hasn't become a dumping ground for old
pill packets, biscuit wrappers and apple cores. I know that
once the space under my bed has gone feral, my sleep goes
haywire. And whilst I don't want to get all feng shui on you, I
actually think a little bit of Japanese culture goes a long way.
They've been practising this stuff for centuries, so although
I'm not suggesting you get a compass out and start being
obsessive about where you put your waste-paper basket, I do
think making your bedroom a serene and comforting space
makes sense.

9. Wind down properly before you attempt to go to bed. Try not
to over-booze, lay off the red wine, but keep yourself hydrated

– chamomile tea is a really good bedtime drink, although many people find something milky like Ovaltine or Horlicks more comforting.

10. I find a nice bath before getting into bed helps enormously. And make sure that whatever you put on to go to bed in, you can whip it off quickly should you feel the dreaded heat surge. The last thing you need to be doing is fighting with buttons.

11. If a hot flush wakes you up, try to keep calm. Don't be tempted to go on Twitter at 3am. In fact, ideally screens should be kept out of the bedroom, because – as we've all been told, countless times – that glowing blue light is really bad for us at night-time. However . . .

12. . . . if it's all getting too much and you're freaking out about never being able to sleep again, distract yourself. In times of great stress and sleeplessness I find an audio book incredibly reassuring. (Make sure you love the narrator's voice though; I once downloaded for my mother Elizabeth Gaskell's *North and South*, which, for some reason, was being read by a shrill American. You could see my mother's hackles rise, every time she turned it on.) There are also lots of brilliant dramas and short stories available for free on the BBC iPlayer (now irritatingly called 'Sounds'), plus there's a world of freebie podcasts, including *Older and Wider*, of course. If audio doesn't work for you, just shut your eyes and rest your body. Tell yourself that this is almost as good as sleep, then indulge in a favourite daydream: take yourself somewhere you know well (this could be a Greek island or your local high street), and once you're in virtual situ, do what you like to do – it might be swimming in the sea, followed by barbecued prawns and a Greek salad,

all washed down with a nice cold glass of retsina, or you might fantasize about buying those shoes you saw the other day in Kurt Geiger, or pony trekking through a nice wood . . . Allow yourself to daydream like you did when you were a kid. Thanks to sleeplessness, over the last few months I've returned to Venice, Morocco and Cornwall; I've also visited the Conran shop and bought all the things I couldn't possibly afford in real life, redesigned my kitchen and built myself a studio in the back garden.

13. And finally, buy a fan – the biggest and blowiest that you can afford. And whatever you do, make sure it's pointing in your direction. Oh – and try and find a quiet one; it's all very well feeling nice and cool, but if it makes more noise than a jet engine about to take off, then it might defeat the object of the exercise.

As with everything during the menopause, the most important thing you can do is to take control of whatever problems you might be experiencing. If sleep deprivation is becoming unbearable, don't just soldier on – talk to your GP. They are highly unlikely to prescribe sleeping pills because that's what they used to do in the old days and a generation of women got hooked on knockout drops for decades (these days, I think only pop stars have the kind of, ahem, doctors that still hand these out), but with any luck, your friendly GP will prescribe something like an anti-histamine which could make you feel drowsy. And, of course, there are plenty of over-the-counter remedies.

For the hot sweats, unless you fancy going down the HRT route (if that's an option for you), then sage is meant to be the miracle herb. If you're not keen on the idea of a sage-tea nightcap, then it's available in tablet form from your local health-food emporium.

Rather than tablets, your GP may recommend sleep therapy, which Podcast Judith attempted with mixed results. Basically, they look at your sleeping habits and try to work out a bedtime timetable, which will encourage your brain and body into a healthier sleep pattern. For Podcast Judith, in order to train her to wake up later, she was instructed to go to bed later which, considering she was used to nodding off during the nine o'clock news, was pretty tricky, as it meant sitting downstairs for two hours yawning before she was 'allowed' to go to bed. In the end, I think the exercise was useful rather than life-transforming.

Isn't it funny – when you were young, the last thing you wanted was to go to bed. Remember all those arguments with your parents about bedtimes? Now, the idea of someone ordering me upstairs on the dot of ten is my idea of heaven. I love my bed, and even on nights when I have trouble getting to sleep (or wake up and can't get back to sleep) I'm still very glad to be in it. I'm comfy and I'm warm – I'm very lucky, really.

OTHER HALVES

'Me and the old man have been together for thirty-seven years – thirty-seven years of sharing the same bed: he has it Mondays, Wednesdays and Fridays.' **JE**

Sometimes I worry this book is a bit heteronormal. But let's be honest here – I'm a straight, white, middle-class woman, living in London with my straight, white husband. There is nothing particularly interesting or unusual about our relationship, unless you count the fact that we have been together for almost forty years (and married for just two).

There are huge numbers of women who are going through the menopause without an 'other half' – and many of these will be going 'solo' by choice. But having someone by your side at this time can be a massive help. As long as that someone isn't a bit of a twat. Imagine that: having to put up with all the hot sweats, brain fog and a massive bloke twat saying the wrong thing and generally being a prick.

There are some men you just know would be rubbish at helping you through the menopause. Fortunately, many of these find the idea so abhorrent they avoid it by marrying much younger women who they get rid of once they start getting a bit chin whiskery and fat around the middle. In my opinion, these men are doing their exes a huge favour.

Older and Wider

Fact: all women who are lucky enough to live long enough will eventually become menopausal; this might be tricky for their other halves to come to terms with but, guess what? We never saw the receding hairline, expanding waistline and nose/ear hair coming either. We never expected to end up with a garden gnome. So let's cut each other some slack here. Growing old is messy for everyone. Most couples are in the same boat and you can either take an oar each and work as a team or get out.

Statistically, there is a proven spike in divorce rates for the over fifties which, I reckon, could be due to one of four reasons:

1. The kids have left home and you have both come to the conclusion that they were the only things you really had in common.
2. He's run off with someone else.
3. You've run off with someone else.
4. The menopause.

Blaming the menopause for the disintegration of a marriage might seem a bit extreme but I can see how it might happen. If a man cannot get his head around what is happening to you and doesn't like the fact that you are a molten bag of fury who doesn't particularly want to have sex, then I reckon you're better off without him. If, however, he thinks you've gone off him because you bite his head off all the time and have taken to sleeping on top of the chest freezer in the garage, then it's possibly time to tell him what's going on before he moves out and you're left feeling more miserable than ever.

Most men in their forties and fifties are quite well sussed these days. They've got the Internet – it's not like the 1950s when a chap didn't really understand what went on in his pretty wife's head, never mind under her frilly nightie.

In years gone by, it was quite common for a woman to get out of bed an hour earlier than necessary in order to put her face on, so her husband never got to see her without her slap. So imagine the lengths she'd have had to go to to hide any evidence of the menopause; imagine being a 1950s housewife and having to pretend to be cheerful and fun, when all you really wanted to do was sit on the sofa and eat cold cauliflower cheese with your fingers.

We've got it made by comparison. Blokes have changed. We've changed. And in any case, pretending things are ok, when they're not is such a waste of everyone's time.

Of course, everyone's relationship with their partner is different. If you're in a same-sex relationship, then bingo – it should be easy: women know what women's bodies do; we know the havoc hormones can cause. But one of the potentially biggest problems in a same-sex, same-age relationship is when you both try to out-menopause each other, with the two of you competing as to who can be the sweatiest bundle of bonkers.

For those of us stuck with menfolk on this adventure through menopause land, then it's only fair we explain that the going could get a little rough, that the terrain might be rocky and that conditions might become arid and uncomfortable for a while. If they still don't get it, then tell it to them straight: 'Now, listen love. I might be a difficult bitch for quite some time and my vagina might feel like the Gobi Desert, but I'm afraid you're going to have to like it or lump it.' At this point, he might do a runner and move in with Linda from the office – but she won't make shepherd's pie like you do and he'll soon see the error of his ways.

If I were writing a guide to the menopause for men – what to expect and how to deal with it – it would be short and to the point:

JENNY ECLAIR'S HANDY BOOK OF TIPS FOR MEN TO HELP THE MRS THROUGH HER MENOPAUSE

1. Don't laugh at her when she is trying to be deadly serious.
2. Don't get embarrassed, even if you are really embarrassed.
3. If you do get embarrassed, have a nice, cold lager, it will stop you blushing whilst she tells you really intimate things about her lady bits.
4. Never paint a window frame so that the window won't open.
5. If you do, don't be surprised when she smashes it open with a shoe.
6. Make sure there is a chilled bottle of something nice in the fridge at all times.
7. Think before you do or say something stupid.
8. Don't compare your mother's menopause to her menopause – i.e. never say, 'Well, my mother says some women just like to make a fuss'.
9. Remember, you are capable of buying lubrication on your own.
10. Don't make jokes about her over the garden fence when you think she's out of earshot. She might be inside the house, but remember every window is now open.

However:

1. Do talk about what's going on with your mates. They might accuse you of having turned into a girl, but it might be a

relief to talk about it with other chaps who are going through the same thing (apart from Roger, of course, who left Mavis for that Russian twenty-six-year-old and is now the father of twins, and consequently hasn't slept since last August bank-holiday Monday and looks like shit. Ha! Remember, guys, there are pros to the menopause.)

2. Do remember to compliment her. Tell her you think she's the bee's knees, that her hair looks nice and that dress really suits her. And, whatever you do, if you accidentally bump into her, look pleased to see her – don't hide in a doorway.

3. Do help. The menopause can have all sorts of different side effects. For example, she might go off cooking, she might suddenly get bored shitless of thinking about what to have for tea every night, especially if she's been doing it for years. Take up some of the slack, do some of the cooking yourself. Because, let's face it, it's the easiest way of getting what you fancy. If you've never done much cooking, look at some cookery books; there are loads of them out there. Word of warning though, if you do get hooked, don't get smug.

4. Encourage her hobbies. Even if you think jigsaws are a waste of time, if it's helping her, then shut it. And don't even think about hiding a piece, so that you can be the one who finishes it.

5. Don't gaslight her. If she is going through a forgetful phase, don't make comments that imply you think she might have early-onset dementia. It's not helpful.

All we really want is someone to make things feel better. Sometimes this can be achieved with something as simple as a cup of tea in bed, a nice (non-gropey) hug, a small bunch of flowers (we don't mind supermarket bouquets, I promise – cheap and cheerful is fine, except when it's a birthday), even a packet of posh sausages or a carefully selected cheese can work wonders. We just want someone who is on our side and will bat for us like they really mean it and won't ever tell us our best dress looks a bit tight.

See – it's not hard, is it? All she needs is for you to behave like a fully grown adult and together you should get through all this.

My partner's biggest mistake is to look really worried if I mention I'm running low on HRT supplies. 'But you will get some more?' he wheedles. And if we're ever packing for a holiday, I know he checks my toiletry bag to make sure I haven't 'forgotten anything' – and I know damn well it's not the blood-pressure medication he's concerned about.

To give men their due, it can't be easy for them to see the woman they love turn into a rabid beast, though how many of us are sweetness and light to begin with I'm not sure.

In my partner's case what unnerved him the most was that I became very weepy and unconfident. He could deal with the swearing and the pot banging, but he didn't know what to do with the new snivelling me; he'd got used to me being a bit gung ho and strident, so it came as a shock when I kept falling to pieces. I reckon that hormone replacement therapy saved not just my sanity, but my career and my relationship. And both of us are just so hugely relieved that it's available and I'm medically compatible with it.

For a lot of couples this can be make-or-break time and I know plenty who have been to marital therapy to help them through it. This is a brilliant idea, because if you can't talk to each other about it, then talking to someone else could make a world of difference. Therapy can work its wonders in all sorts of ways. A couple of friends of mine went and suddenly found themselves agreeing on something for the first time in years. Ok, so it's a shame the thing they found themselves agreeing on was that they both thought their counsellor was a knobhead, but that's beside the point; it got them agreeing, it got them laughing and the next thing they knew they were in the pub sharing a bag of dry-roasted. And five years later they're still together. See!

So don't rule anything out. All relationships can have rough patches and often it's not just the menopause that's making things tough. There's all the other midlife crap that's going on as well – family stuff, work stuff, money stuff – and sometimes we start behaving badly to the person who's closest because we just need someone to blame, even if it's completely irrational.

Fear of the future can be one of the menopause's sneaky side effects. Let's just shove this one under the umbrella of 'general anxiety'. I remember getting very gloomy about entering the next stage of my life and I'm grateful to have the old man's hand to hold, even if it's less of a hand than a paw; my husband has the mitts of a mature grizzly bear, but there is something very reassuring about them, especially when he gives my hand a squeeze back and says, 'It'll be alright, porker.'

And who knows? It just might be.

JOINT MENOPAUSE SURVIVAL GUIDE

1. Do share the remote control, I'm not saying put a timer on the thing, but actually, that's not a bad idea. Here's how it works in our house: because I watch less telly on the whole than my partner, I get to choose the 9pm to 10pm sweet viewing spot. Sometimes, when there's nothing decent on, we go over to Netflix and by the time we've found something we both fancy, it's ten o'clock, my time slot is over and, in any case, we're both so knackered, it's time to go to bed.

2. If insomnia and night sweats are causing havoc in the bedroom, try a joint audio book. Several months ago, when I was going through a lousy sleeping phase, we found that being read to on a nightly basis really helped. Choosing something you're both going to like is a great opportunity to broaden your reading horizons. Over the past couple of years, we've both listened to books we probably wouldn't have chosen just for ourselves. I think this is how compromise works!

3. Try and find a joint hobby – something that you actually enjoy doing together, now you can't be arsed with sex any more. Of course, for couples who are still happily banging away, then you don't need to bother; for the rest of us – why do you think they invented garden centres?

P

PERIODS

'I can't see the point in having periods when you're really old. You'd be forever forgetting to put a tampon in and leaving a trail of blood all the way to the post office (which is one way of finding your way home, I suppose).' **JE**

Many people think that the menopause is first and foremost about periods, and it's true that a woman is medically menopausal when she ceases to menstruate regularly. But as we all know, it's a great deal more complicated than no longer losing a few tablespoons of blood every month.

That said, periods are a huge part of a woman's life and every woman's cycle is completely different. Some will rarely have experienced menstruation, whilst for others it can be the bane of their lives, but either way, bleeding too much or too little can cause both physical and mental pain.

For the majority of us, blood in our knickers is just one of the rites of womanhood. It's weird when it starts, but it's equally weird when it stops and you realize that instead of pushing your trolley down the feminine-hygiene aisle, you're heading straight to bin liners and cat food.

IN THE BEGINNING

I started my periods when I was fourteen, which was quite late, even back in the 1970s.

At the time, I was very eager to experience the phenomenon. I wanted the excuse to get out of games at school and go running off to matron for a couple of aspirin and a lie down in the san; I wanted to use one of those paper bags that hung on the back of toilet doors with the picture of the lady in a crinoline on the front. (What was that all about? By the time I was twelve I had it figured out – possibly the crinolined lady was symbolic of all menstruating women, what with her being in period dress?! And so went my first period gag.)

The reality of my first period wasn't quite so hilarious though. I was wearing a pair of pink Bri-Nylon pyjamas and woke up around 5am to find them sticky with blood. My mother, who I decided must be alerted to this drama, rolled out of bed, chucked a box of Dr Whites at me and muttered, 'Oh poor you, another forty years of this.' Thirty-eight as it happened.

I was of the generation lucky enough to begin my relationship with feminine-hygiene products with the stick-on pads that adhered to the gusset of one's knickers. These were a bit chunky, but much less bulky than the previous generation of massive thick cotton pads that came with a plastic belt, loops and safety pins and made anyone wearing them walk like they were in nappies.

Obviously, after a few months of dealing with the boring, 'no-swim-ming' towel option, I decided to try tampons, desperately attempting to insert one by jabbing at my vagina with that cardboard tube, slavishly copying the diagram, foot up on the lavatory seat. Maybe because I'd been a keen young pony rider, I eventually emerged, tampon successfully inserted (with just a bit hanging out), cantering triumphantly from the bathroom. But it was ages until I managed to figure out the angle of my cervix and pop them in without looking.

From then on, my period was just a monthly bore, although not being a clockwork type kept me on my toes and I was occasionally caught off guard throughout my teens, leading to those horrified scuttles to the nearest bathroom, convinced that the back of my skirt would be stained and wondering if I could actually die of embarrassment.

But to be fair, I didn't suffer with my periods as much as some of the girls in my year. I wasn't a puker or a fainter. And even if I had been, my mother belonged to the school of mothering that believed a good, brisk cycle ride was the answer to all ills – and that included period pains.

THE PERIOD-FREE ANOREXIC YEARS

I did have a prolonged period holiday when, for several years, I was bleed-free and, at the time, I spent the tampon money on fags. This hiatus began at drama school when, thanks mostly to the staff instilling in me a phobia of being the 'fat actress who never gets any work', I managed to whittle myself down to just under seven stone.

I was nineteen when I started dieting, having already weathered a year of jibes from one particular tutor (which would quite rightly constitute a sacking offence now). At the time, I was probably a chunky size twelve, possibly verging on a fourteen – so not fat-fat, but borderline to a critical eye.

I'd been plump as a schoolgirl, but not disastrously so; my mother was a good cook, but encouraged me to be sensible. Back in the 1970s, mothers tended to be vigilant about their daughters' weight and mine occasionally encouraged me to 'cut back a bit'.

What can I say? I was a very greedy girl. My favourite thing was waking up to an empty house, cooking myself a full English, scoffing the lot and then repeating the process.

We lived in a roomy detached Victorian house with a large walk-in pantry and my mother baked. This was a lethal combination. Sometimes I'd come home from school and do a circuit of the cake tins. I'd shut the door, then, armed with a sharp knife, I'd start hacking at fruit cake, neatening off Victoria sponges and filling my pockets with something my mother called 'chocolate biscuit cake'. (This was a traybake concoction of crushed digestive biscuits, smashed together with syrup, then covered in cooking chocolate and left to set in the fridge.)

I liked cold meats and cheeses too. Oooh, and crisps – I loved a big fistful of nuts and crisps. And I was sly: the kind of girl who pretended to be helping with the dishes, so that I could stuff myself with leftovers – cold roast potatoes, that sticky bit of glazed ham, one last mouthful of trifle . . .

My mother was in hospital the summer I was nineteen. I can't remember now what was wrong with her (which says a great deal about both of us; I was hideously self-absorbed and she has always been stoic to the point of negligence) – she may even have been having a kidney removed? Whatever, she wasn't around for several weeks and I returned home from Manchester to 'look after' my father and much younger brother. This was when I embarked on my 'serious diet'. With no one filling the cake tins, I was mostly cooking mince dishes and, whilst I served my Bologneses with pasta and my chillis with rice for my dad and Ben, I restricted myself to a smear of meat sauce on a chopped-up lettuce or cabbage base. The menfolk didn't notice and my mother wasn't around to question what was going on. It was weirdly easy.

At lunchtime, having made sandwiches for the boys, I sipped a mug of low-cal soup, stopped eating buttered toast and switched to Ryvita. Breakfast, meanwhile, consisted of a great deal of fruit and just a little natural yoghurt.

Exercise wasn't a big deal in those days, so I didn't bother with that. I just cut down the calories and fell in love with the results. Oh, hello, cheekbones. Hello, tiny waist and clavicles.

Back at drama school for the beginning of my second year, people marvelled at my transformation. All of a sudden, I felt like one of the cute ones. My jeans fell off me, I wore bright yellow Anello & Davide dance shoes and a yellow sweatshirt. I felt great.

But my flatmate, 'beautiful Frances', eyed me warily.

Suddenly, we weren't sharing meals any more. Within weeks I'd cut my breakfast down to artificially sweetened stewed apple, flavoured with cinnamon, lunch was my usual low-cal cuppa soup and by now, supper was more low-cal soup with extra veg thrown in (beansprouts bulked everything out). I would take an hour to eat under 200 calories and any snacks consisted of oranges or raw carrots dipped in Marmite.

Frances, with her milkmaid curves, got really fed up, and in an effort to make me eat a proper meal, invited some of our year round for a big lasagne. Obviously, I made excuses, pretending to have turned veggie, so she cooked me some veg instead, but when I saw her put butter in the pan, I had a complete meltdown and threw the butter out of the window. Then, when she screamed that she couldn't afford to waste butter on a student grant, I promptly climbed out of the kitchen window and started crawling across the roof to fetch it back.

Food was going to kill me, one way or another.

By the time I was in my third year, keeping my weight down had taken priority over everything else. College was a mere distraction. I wasn't even bothering with men any more, which, considering I'd been a bit of a slag since my mid-teens, was completely out of character. I took the odd line of coke, went out, got pissed and came home. I was too tired for sex and anyway, the weight of someone else on top of me became uncomfortable. I didn't really have the strength for it. Frances was by now eating chocolate bars in the toilet. I used to find the wrappers and think, Greedy cow. In the end, she'd had enough and grassed me up to the college. I should have thanked her but I was livid.

My mother was alerted to the situation and came up with my aunt. The two of them, in their good jackets and pleated skirts, took me out for lunch and I pretended to eat. By this point my cunning was pretty impressive.

They went home reassured that I wasn't going to be 'silly' any more. Ha, the fools! I continued to lose weight – every spare ounce that I could, every inch of fat. Once the flesh was gone and I was down to my barest bones, I grazed my spine sliding down in the bath, and in the months that followed, I developed a soft, downy pelt of fine hair all over – my body was desperately trying to protect itself, the soft down being a weirdly primitive way of keeping me warm enough to survive (we're more animal than we like to think).

College called me in, threats were made, I was frogmarched to a counsellor, he was useless and I bailed out of college in the final term, too weak to finish the course.

My periods had stopped sometime the previous year, although I hadn't really noticed. Everything was shutting down. I went home and tried to sort it all out without actually putting any weight back on and the battle continued.

In the end, I was anorexic for around five years. I got better very gradually (a little bit of therapy, sadly in the wrong hands, didn't help), eventually boring myself out of the disease – it had controlled my life for too long and I'd had enough. My partner (now husband) was endlessly patient, paying bills in restaurants, even when I'd ordered and bolted. My recovery was steady but slow, and I didn't have another period until I was twenty-five. I remember it well – I got caught out in a pair of tartan trousers. They were wool and I could never quite get the surprise-surprise stain out of the gusset.

Of course, three years later they stopped again. Only then it was because I was pregnant.

I was very lucky to have a child. With my history, I could have damaged my fertility beyond repair. So, whilst I never welcomed my periods with open arms, I knew that their continuing arrival meant that everything was in working order and that the anorexia was a thing of the past.

After the birth of my first and only child, I had another couple of decades of regular-ish periods, although – unless I was on the Pill – I was never a woman who came on every twenty-eight days. My cycle was rather longer, averaging around thirty-two days (nothing is ever 100 per cent science, is it?). And I always knew when I was due on because I'd have two days of extreme lethargy, weepiness and lack of confidence, followed by the arrival of my period, heralding a sudden turbo-charged surge in both mental and physical strength. This would last for several days before dwindling throughout the remainder of the month, until, once again, I was a cringing, neurotic mess. I'm sure most women feel this hormonal ebb and flow of confidence. It's infuriating because at times it seems like one's career has been ruled entirely by the thinning and thickening of one's womb lining!

THE PERI-MENOPAUSE

According to my mother, the peri-menopause is quite a newfangled thing. My grandmother certainly didn't have one, although she did get her bosom caught in the mangle, so you know, swings and round-abouts!

The peri-menopause is a kind of phoney menopause. It's the warm-up act before the show really begins. Basically, it means you will feel a bit menopausal now and again, you might have the occasional hot flush and your periods will start acting up, eventually becoming less reliable than Network Rail.

Just to warn you: when your periods are on the wane due to the approaching menopause, do not be surprised if they suddenly become horrifically heavy, monstrously clotty and last for weeks on end. However, don't take my word on this; for heaven's sake, speak to your doctor – because what's normal for one woman isn't necessarily normal for another, and no one should ever feel they are wasting anyone's time when it comes to matters gynae. So if in doubt – see the doctor. And, by the way, just because your ovaries may have shut up shop, it doesn't mean you can stop going for smear tests. Lie back on that paper sheet, spread those knees and thank the NHS for trying to keep women as safe as possible.

PS Most women will experience the menopause between the ages of forty-five and fifty-five; some will go through it much earlier, due to premature ovarian insufficiency or other reasons, sometimes unknown, but the average age in the UK is fifty-one, so at fifty-two, I was only a year out!

I talked to my ninety-year-old mother about her menopause. She was slightly vague about it. She said, 'That sort of thing wasn't very fashionable back in the early 1980s, unlike now when it seems all the rage.' The only thing she could remember was finishing her periods when she was fifty-two and thinking no more about them until a year later when she went into hospital for an operation, only to start a period completely out of the blue as she was being wheeled to the operating room. She said everyone was really cross with her. Like it was my poor old mum's fault.

AWFUL PERIOD-RELATED DISASTERS

When I was at drama school, I did a short run of a Theatre in Education play, for school children. The contents of the script are hazy – it was probably about road safety or not talking to strangers or just saying 'No' to drugs – and all I can remember is that I was playing an acrobatic clown (listen, I could cartwheel back then) and white satin trousers were involved. And yup, you guessed it, ten minutes after I cartwheeled onstage I came on like a geyser and for the rest of the show I was cartwheeling with firmly closed legs. ('Didn't think much of the acrobatic clown,' came the muttered playground review.)

Another time, onstage at the Edinburgh Festival, my tampon came out. I was wearing tight, stretchy bell-bottom leggings and no pants, so I had to leave the stage and re-insert the damn thing before it could fall out the bottom of the leggings and roll into the front row. Once back onstage, I couldn't come up with any reason for having left my audience so abruptly, so I told them the truth, which was met by a sort of horrified silence.

Back in the 1990s I was in a West End stage production of *Steaming*, a play written by Nell Dunn, which was set in a Turkish bath house and thus featured a fantastic, fully functioning on-set swimming pool. One night, I divebombed into said pool slightly too enthusiastically during the curtain call and lost my tampon, whereupon the actress Julie T. Wallace insisted I go back onstage after the audience had left the auditorium and fish it out, which I dutifully did!

AN APOLOGY

I would like to end this chapter with an apology to all those hotels and B&Bs up and down the country where I lost track of the dates and came on in the middle of the night. Oh no, what to do? I never knew whether or not to try and scrub the stain out, inevitably leaving a massive great pink damp patch and the hotel staff concluding that not only had I bled all over the sheets, but I'd wet the bed too.

Messy business being a girl.

See? It's a great relief to be old enough not to worry about such things. Mind you, these days, when I fart onstage, I always have a tiny panic that I might have shat myself. We only ever really swap one problem for another.

QUALITY QUICHE

'I know I've changed because my partner bought me an oven glove for my birthday, and I didn't immediately want to divorce him.' **JE**

I have never been a baker. Some women are born with pastry-making hands. Not me. I'm a complete novice in the kitchen. At fifty-nine, I have the cooking skills of a teenager – but I'm not as bad as I used to be because, oddly enough, the menopause, with all its peculiar side effects, has ignited a small pilot light in my heart for cooking.

Now whether this means watching other people do it, having a go myself or scoffing the results, I'm all for learning how to eat better and cheaper in my own home and I am now the proud owner of about six recipe books!

In my defence, one of the reasons why I have such poor cooking skills is that, thanks to stand-up, I have spent a huge amount of time on the road. It's very difficult to prepare a fantastic evening meal whilst you're halfway up the M6 on your way to do a gig in Carlisle.

For years, my culinary speciality was sandwiches, but boy, was I good with sandwiches! I'd say for about twenty years, most of the meals produced in my house were shoved between two slices of bread. Sometimes I'd make a sandwich from the remains of the previous night's Indian takeaway and eat that for breakfast. It's only because I had help looking after my daughter that she avoided rickets. As it was, she was seven before she had enough strength in her legs to be able to pedal a bike; I thought she had coordination problems, but the doctor just said she was rather 'weak'. This was my fault entirely.

I once lived in a house with no oven for a number of years. I had a hob and a microwave – what did I need an oven for? It was only when I realized that you physically can't microwave a full Christmas dinner for an entire family of twelve that I relented and had an oven installed. It was either a new Neff or turkey nuggets for twelve.

It's taken me a long time to 'get' cooking – to realize that actually being able to feed your family from scratch is cool. That said, I'm still not a baker. The truth is I haven't made a cake since I left school.*

I love cooking programmes. For some reason, I find them incredibly calming. In fact, I frequently find myself watching people create the most spectacular things in spun sugar and meringue, whilst balancing a ready meal on my lap. I'm a big fan of medicinal telly, and whilst nothing has tempted me to buy specialist confectionery gear yet (to me, the '20-hole reinforced silicone cake popper' sounds like something you might get from a fetish shop), over the past few years, I have found myself happily messing around on the nursery slopes of cooking. I started by making soup, which led to casseroles,

---

* **CORRECTION** I *hadn't* baked a cake since school until I was asked (out of the blue) to be a contestant on Channel 4's 2020 *Great Celebrity Bake Off* for *Stand Up to Cancer*. I had precisely one day to practise a biscuit recipe and my non-existent choux pastry skills, both of which were a disaster, and I entered that *Bake Off* tent with a heavy heart. If you want to see the results, I'm sure there's a YouTube clip or two online. All I'm going to say is that I've still got the pinny!

which led to stir-fries and now I find myself doing something quite daring about three times a week. This is progress for me.

In some respects, it's not about the results. It's about reconnecting with something that I lost touch with many years ago.

Convenience foods are all very well, but making a meal with fresh ingredients has a sort of authenticity that I want in my life right now. There is something a bit silly about being a menopausal woman who cannot cook at all. It's naff not being able to throw a few basic dishes together, although, sadly, my boring tomato allergy rules out all the really easy mince staples.

In any case, I've run out of excuses. I'm not on the road as much as I used to be, and these days there are months of being at home, writing, writing, writing. Who'd have known that chopping vegetables could be so therapeutic? Apart from the butternut squash, of course. That's not therapeutic – that's a workout and dangerous too. In fact, every butternut squash should come with a health-and-safety label: 'Warning! Cutting this up could lead to a trip to A&E.'

There is a certain pride that comes with cooking. And it's also a generous thing. I have a neighbour in her sixties who repays even the tiniest favour in plates of buns, fairy cakes or biscuits. To be able to do something like this is such a great life skill and surely just as valuable as being able to apply a really great smoky eye or a massively painted-on eyebrow.

I think anything that helps menopausal women get through what can be a mentally challenging time is worth its weight in dirty pans. If you're feeling a bit down, trying a new recipe can be almost as satisfying as buying a new pair of shoes, but without the hefty price tag. Cooking is alchemy: you bundle a load of bits and bobs together and hey presto (or possibly pesto), sometime later something that smells and tastes delicious emerges from the oven ready to be shared (or not).

I think a lot of us have fallen out of love with the ready-made. I'm not saying we're turning our backs on convenience foods entirely, but I know I'm putting slightly less pre-packaged stuff into my trolley and lobbing in a lot more raw ingredients. Homemade is back in, thanks to the popularity of programmes such as *Masterchef* and *Bake Off*. And wonky cakes and burned crusts are a sign of not being mass produced. Seriously, I made cauliflower cheese for the first time in my life last year and my heart almost burst with pride. Was it as good as Marks's? No, but I got twice as much for half the price – and yes, cauliflower cheese does freeze.

For women, particularly of my generation, reclaiming the kitchen is something that feels strangely powerful, which is odd, when it should be against all our feminist principles. After all, we were the generation who turned our backs on domesticity and yet, here we are, tying pinnies around our waists completely by choice.

I think what the menopause does is bring us to a point of crux. There's no going back. We are entering a truly adult stage of our lives – one where we're still fit, still *compos mentis* and still have everything going for us. It's a time when it feels really important to make some decisions about how we want to live from now on. We aren't girls anymore; we're women. By now, we should be free of all that crippling self-consciousness and the career doubts that plagued us when we were younger. We might not be able to change the world, but we can change how we live in the world. We can decide that what we want is some real quality in our lives, and if this means covering our hands with flour and rolling out a quiche base, then so be it. Who knows how much time we have left, so why not spend as much of that time as possible doing things that a) we enjoy and b) we can feel proud of – whether that's bungee jumping or Victoria sponge baking, it doesn't matter. It's about a sense of achievement.

There's also possibly a bit of nostalgia mixed in with my new-found appreciation for kitchen DIY. Even though she's still very much alive and cooking, there is something about my mother's handwriting in an old recipe book that tugs on my heart strings. It reminds me of when I was young. I come from a world of the homemade. My mother wouldn't have dreamed of buying me a birthday cake; in any case, my parties predated shop-bought novelty cakes, and back in the 1960s you couldn't get cake tins in anything other than round, square or oblong. Hence, my birthday cake was always some variation of a Victoria sponge, often with those tiny decorative teeth-shattering silver balls scattered on top. Now that was sophistication.

Why Quiche?

Whilst I'm not interested in cakes, I do want to conquer the quiche, even if it means beginning with shop-bought pastry. (The way I see it, as long as it's hand-crimped in the dish, it still counts as homemade!)

The homemade quiche (even when the pastry is both soggy *and* dry) is somehow redolent of honesty and a lack of pretention. It reminds me of visits to wine bars in the 1970s, way back when it was as newfangled as sushi. It's a memory of picnics eaten on red tartan rugs on beaches with rock pools that turned your toes blue. It's sort of symbolic of lots of things the menopausal woman finds herself attracted to . . .

I like a village fete, a brass band playing in a park pavilion, ice-cream van music, ducks on a pond and a cream tea on the end of a pier, parks with cafes serving misshapen scones and soup that doesn't come out of a packet; I like my chips big and chunky from a proper fish and chippy; biscuit tins with pictures of dogs on them and brightly coloured seersucker tablecloths; and, yes, I like bunting and old-fashioned (non-helium) balloons and small jugs of freshly cut flowers, all higgledy-piggledy as table decorations.

And I like quiche.

Of course, even better than knowing what you like is knowing what you don't like.

I don't like butter in stupid little foil pats and piddling sachets of sauces. I want my ketchup, mayo and mustard in big bottles on the table, please.

I don't like big telly screens in pubs, especially when they are automatically tuned to sports channels, featuring blokes playing football, when the only punters are three women, who would rather change channels but aren't allowed.

I don't like children watching cartoons on iPads in smart restaurants after 9pm without headphones; or silly amuse-bouche courses which involve wafer-thin cut radish or a foam of something that looks like a toad coughed on your plate.

I don't like being asked my name in a coffee shop, only for them to misspell it on a paper cup.

I don't like hotels which serve hot food that's been stewed in troughs for hours under horrible bright lights.

I don't like fake flowers when the real versions are in season, especially when the fake ones are so realistic that you feel a fool when you finally realize they're fabric. I especially hate those.

I want things simple. I want things real. I'm sick of fake. I don't like acrylic fingernails or hair extensions that are all maggoty at the roots.

I feel sad about fake tits and blown-up lips and hairless pudendas. I want pants that can contain my bottom and a bra that doesn't dig in and I want pockets everywhere and a bag that zips up easily that can comfortably hold everything – just like my pants.

Which brings me to my next point, the wonderful thing about being of menopausal age is that we are no longer beholden to fashion. Fashion isn't interested in us (despite the fact that our demographic has more money than most), so why should we be interested in trends? I don't want my gin flavoured with mint and chocolate, but I do want it clean and sharp in a proper glass that isn't still hot from the dishwasher behind the bar. We are now of an age when we're not prepared to compromise. For me, this means sending food back if it's not up to standard, asking people in the quiet coach to *be* quiet and to move rooms in hotels if mine smells weird or is next to a clanking lift.

Being a menopausal woman also gives me the right to tell grown men off for cycling on the pavement, to shove litter back in someone's hand and to turn off that TV programme that everyone else is raving about but which I can't stand.

We might as well start pleasing ourselves at this stage in our lives and that's why it's really important to know what makes us tick more happily as time goes by. As a feminist, it seems odd to be suggesting we get back in the kitchen, but I genuinely believe that anything that distracts us, saves money and gives us a sense of pride really helps with dealing with the menopausal down days, and if that involves sticking more buns in the oven, then so be it. At least this lot won't need shoes!

R

REMEDIES

'One woman's black cohosh is another woman's Blue Nun.' JE

There are as many remedies for the menopause as there are symptoms – in other words, a lot.

HORMONE REPLACEMENT THERAPY (HRT)

Let's start with the ultimate avoidance tactic – hormone replacement therapy – which basically sidesteps many menopausal miseries and yet is still the subject of much controversy. For example, there are some people (e.g. my sister) who genuinely believe HRT is the wuss's way out and that in some weird moral way, it's cheating!

Now just hold on a minute . . . For one thing, I never expected to resort to HRT. I always thought I'd get through the menopause like my mother did – on cooking sherry and biscuits. But as I've already explained in this book: needs must. For me, it was either HRT or Holloway (which, sadly for this joke, has actually closed down) and I've never regretted my choice.

As I also mentioned earlier in the book, for the past seven years, I've been on a daily pill plus a rub-in gel combination, Noriday and Oestrogel (AKA mother's little helpers). Oestrogel comes in a pump-action bottle that squirts a see-through substance that feels a little bit like congealing sperm against the skin, but don't let that put you off!

I'm on two pumps a day, which I rub into my upper left shoulder. Alternatively, it can be rubbed into the inside of one's thigh (for extra kicks). This seems ridiculous, but I believe the way it works is that the oestrogen in the gel is absorbed through the skin into the bloodstream. Honestly, medicine can be quite magical sometimes.

HRT has been around since the 1940s but due to continued fears over potential health risks many women are switching to . . .

. . . BIOIDENTICAL HORMONE THERAPY (BHT)

BHT is gradually becoming more popular for women who have decided they need hormone replacement but would rather keep things more natural.

Now that it's no longer made from the urine of pregnant horses, normal HRT is made from synthetic hormones. BHT uses plant oestrogens that identically chemically match the hormones our bodies produce naturally. And you know, if I was just setting out on my menopause hike now, this is probably the option I'd be looking at. That said, according to research, there is no concrete evidence that BHT is any more effective or any safer than your bog-standard HRT. As ever, the choice is yours.

Of course, for some women, hormone replacement therapy is not an option in any form. This might be due to medical circumstances or personal belief. So what other remedies are there?

DIET

I have a thirty-year-old daughter who is incredibly vigilant about managing her health and allergy issues by controlling her diet. Hence, she is dairy, soya and gluten free. But she's a lot more disciplined than me and I doubt that I could create and stick to a diet that could adequately manage my menopausal symptoms without any other sort of help.

This isn't to say that I sneer at the idea of a menopause-friendly diet. I think anything that works and makes us healthier and happier is essentially what we're all after. However, for those of us who aren't trained nutritionists and can't afford to go and see one, the online diet advice for menopausal women seems both annoyingly vague and irritatingly obvious. The general note seems to be: lots of veg and fruit, whole grains and dairy (unless you're lactose intolerant), cutting down on saturated fats and swapping them for unsaturated fats (I think we got that memo years ago) and that age-old adage of plenty of oily fish to top up your omega 3 levels. All this sounds like common sense to me, but anything more specific is trickier to pin down.

For most of us, finding a diet that suits us can be a case of trial and error. When I was peri-menopausal in my late forties, I developed lots of tiny painful ulcers around my gums and on my tongue. Sometimes these would grow in clusters and join up to create one massive, agonizing bleeding sore. My doctor and dentist didn't have any answers; blood tests were taken but the results were inconclusive, and my doctor talked vaguely about it being hormonal but was reluctant to commit to any particular diagnosis. All I know for certain is that it was only through trawling the Internet and visiting lots of mouth-ulcer forums that I gathered that red fruits, especially tomatoes, could often trigger these outbreaks. Consequently, it's been a decade since I last ate any seeded red fruits, including raspberries and strawberries (although watermelon is fine). The things I miss most though are tomatoes (raw or cooked), but on reflection, they were definitely the worst offenders.

Life is a great deal duller without tomatoes in my life. I can't tell you how often I crave a meaty red spaghetti Bolognese, ratatouille or even good old beans on toast. But sadly, I can't even go near a dollop of ketchup. This means a great deal of careful label reading (cue glasses perched on top of head and lots of squinting in the supermarket) because tomatoes, particularly in the form of purée or powder, sneak into everything. All this is very tedious, but very necessary, as the alternative really hurts and makes it difficult to speak which, as you can imagine, is tricky in my line of work.

I still get the occasional mouth ulcer but by keeping my diet free from all these delicious red treats I can keep them under control. Prevention is always best, particularly when there is no real cure.

So I know from personal experience that tweaking your life style can improve your health, but it's a huge topic to cover and so, as I'm no expert, let's just agree on a few basic rules:

- Don't just sit around eating rubbish.
- Cut down on the booze.

- And if you're still doing it, for heaven's sake . . . quit smoking – it's a killer. I gave up around fifteen years ago with the aid of nicotine patches, and I promise you, if I can give up, anyone can.

BOOZE

Cutting down on the booze is easier said than done. Never mind those unit reminders on the backs of bottles, we might all go a bit easier on the stuff if we knew how many extra calories we were chucking down our necks every night.

Alcohol is sadly not a remedy. Oh that it were. Unfortunately, it's full of empty calories which will cause havoc with your weight. It will also make you aggressive, argumentative and in danger of repeating yourself. Your skin will redden and coarsen and you will get big booze pouches under your eyes. Also, because it weakens your resolve, you will find that whilst you're drinking you are also knocking back the nuts and crisps. And so it continues.

Still, it's nice to take the edge off the day now and then, though increasingly I've found that anything over two large glasses makes me feel like I've been in a mystery car crash. Tut. And I used to be so good at drinking.

RECREATIONAL DRUGS

Whilst I'm still a pushover for my nightly Chardonnay fix, I did manage to give up all recreational drugs years ago. I'm sorry, but a fifty-plus-year-old woman who is still doing coke is probably an addict and needs help. Ditto ecstasy, ketamine or anything else that I'm too uncool to know about.

NATURAL REMEDIES

Although I have chosen to go down the chemical route to deal with my menopause, I am certainly not averse to more natural alternatives. The most popular herbal relief remedies for the menopause include the following plants, most of which naturally contain the holy grail of the menopausal woman – oestrogen:

- Red clover – an attractive herbaceous perennial which also causes horses to slobber excessively.
- Black cohosh – a pretty woodland flowering plant belonging to the same family as the buttercup.
- Dong quai – officially classified as belonging to the wild celery family.
- Ginseng – a Chinese root long known to increase libido.
- Kava – not the booze one, this kava is made from the root of a pepper plant species.
- Evening primrose oil – possibly the most famous of all herbal remedies, over the years it's been used to cure everything from skin disorders to PMT and, of course, the menopause. Extracting your own oil from evening primroses is apparently almost impossible; however, the oily seeds can be sprinkled into salads and mixed into smoothies.
- Sea buckthorn oil – this is rich in fatty acids which appar-

ently maintain healthy cell barriers and regular use is said to reverse vaginal atrophy and help with the itching. This can be especially useful for women who can't use oestrogen creams or suppositories.

Most herbal treatments are available in supplement form but some, like sea buckthorn, can be applied directly to the skin. For further information and help on all the natural remedies available, visit your local Holland and Barrett. (Alternatively, wouldn't it be wonderful if you could grow your own herbal menopause window box? They should sell them as kits on Amazon.)

A QUICK DIY PICK-ME-UP

I haven't tried this myself but apparently sage is great for reducing both mood swings and hot flushes. Although it's available as a supplement in tablet form, you might like to make a tea using sage leaves. And any leftovers can be added to breadcrumbs and an onion and used to stuff a chicken. Now if a nice roast dinner doesn't make you feel better, then there's no helping you.

ACUPUNCTURE

Although I control my menopause symptoms with drugs, I'm a big fan of acupuncture and have used it for various other reasons, mostly for anxiety and stress. I'm very fortunate to have found a genius acupuncturist locally who uses a heated acupuncture table. I cannot tell you how many times I have nodded off on this table whilst covered in pins, nor can I describe the miracles she has managed to perform. A lot of people are very cynical about acupuncture – most of these people have never even tried it. The problem is that it's not usually something that you can expect to get on the National Health and therefore it's often a pricey private option.

However, if you're lucky enough to be able to afford it, a small study recently published in the *BMJ* suggested that acupuncture to treat menopausal symptoms might be worth considering. The Danish study found that five weeks of regular treatment was enough to reduce both physical and emotional problems associated with the menopause, and I for one would endorse that.

MAGNETS IN YOUR PANTS

This, on the other hand, is something that makes my bullshit detector twitch, although obviously I'd be happy to be proved wrong.

Magnetic therapy is a slightly bewildering world. The magnets might be integrated into bracelets, rings, anklets and shoe inserts. For true believers, therapeutic magnetic mattresses are also available. Now usually, I'm not one to pooh-pooh anything I've not tried, but I have to say I draw the line at sticking a magnet in my knickers. But for those who are willing to try anything, the market leader the LadyCare Plus Magnet purports to work by rebalancing your autonomic nervous system (ANS), which is the part of the nervous system that's involuntary. According to a magazine article about the magic magnet in *Woman & Home*:

More precisely, it's said to reduce excessive sympathetic nervous system (SNS) activity and increase parasympathetic nervous system (PNS) activity. The SNS and PNS work together to regulate the activity of every organ system in the human body. However, hormonal changes around the time of the menopause can affect their equilibrium, causing SNS activity to increase at the expense of PNS activity.

Sorry but I zoned out halfway through that explanation because I don't actually understand any of it. Oh, listen – you're either going to believe in this kind of thing or you'll be rolling your eyeballs at the idea.

Warning: I once talked to a female teacher who said that because of the magnets in her knickers she was able to control the opening and shutting of the fire doors in her school corridors. Now, if this is true, sign me up! Imagine – it would be like having a superpower in your pants.

CRYSTALS

For those of us who don't want to find ourselves irresistibly drawn to our supermarket trolleys because of our magnetic pants, then there's always crystals.

Ok, I remember crystals being quite big in the 1980s, but it seems they never really went away, and for anyone who still believes, a handy velvet pouch of menopause-healing crystals can be purchased on the Internet for just a few quid. These might contain a mixture of any of the following: fire agate, smoky quartz, lapis lazuli, moonstone, labradorite, rhodonite and chrysoprase.

According to the advertising blurb, 'These precious healing stones can be carried around in the bag or worn discreetly next to the skin.'

Yeah, whatever. At this point, the cynical voice in my head starts muttering, 'We're not in California, love. It's a Tuesday afternoon in south London and it's pissing down. Let's get real.' Meanwhile, the superstitious, more gullible voice in my head mutters, 'Well, you never know . . . ' Only I think I do!

Ok, here's the bottom line girls, we all have our own faiths and beliefs and whatever gets you through the day – as long as it's not illegal or hurting anyone else – is absolutely cool with me. However unusual your coping mechanism is, if it works for you, don't let me be the one to put you off.

S

SANDWICH GENERATION

'Not only are we menopausal, we're suddenly part of the sandwich generation too – squashed on one side by aged parents who are forever tripping up over the carpet and ending up in A&E (200 miles away) and needy kids on the other who can't afford their own mortgages let alone chip in to pay off yours.' **JE**

One of the interesting things about the menopause is how different it is for each individual woman. Some experience years of mayhem and misery, whilst others have one hot flush and bingo, that's them done and dusted.

But I don't think it's just the menopause that is causing all the chaos for many of us. I think the Big M is just one of the many symptoms of suddenly finding yourself middle-aged. Because even if you have a plain-sailing menopause, there are other issues at play. You are in the eye of the storm, lady.

For most middle-aged women there's a great deal of other life crap going on, and for some reason, society expects us to cope with it all. I don't know who coined the phrase 'the sandwich generation', but for many of us it's painfully apt because we are the ones stuck between parents on one side and kids on the other, desperately trying to hold everything together.

Our mums and dads are suddenly getting old, ill and even dying (how dare they, that wasn't part of the deal, they promised to look after us forever). And whilst it's all mobility aids and grab bars on one side, on the other those chubby pink-toed babies you once held in the crook of your arm are leaving home without a backward glance. Or not, as the case might be . . . because for many menopausal women, especially those who live in London, just when you think you're done with the mothering, they come boomeranging back, eating all the cereal and pinching your best cashmere jumper. The only solution to this re-nesting dilemma is to downsize radically, but as we all know, moving is one of the most stressful things you can do in life and moving on top of the menopause is a potentially lethal combination.

Ditto divorce. You might hate each other's guts at the moment, but just give it a couple of years and then, if you still can't bear the sight of each other, maybe it's time to call it a day. All I'm saying is just don't do anything rash whilst your oestrogen levels are plummeting through the floor – try not to make life any harder than it already is. That said, loads of my mates have gone through the menopause as single women, and whilst some would have quite liked a mate cheering them on from the sidelines, others were just glad there wasn't yet more body heat adding to the nightly inferno of bedtime.

As we all know, divorce is a fact of life and more couples are doing it later in life than ever before. No one takes the break-up of a relationship lightly, especially a long-term partnership involving years of building homes and families together. But it does happen, and how you feel about it will depend on whether the break-up is amicable or toxic and what kind of circumstances you find yourself in afterwards. I've seen friends split up well and I've seen friends split up badly; most manage something in between, but, however well you cope with it, there's no guarantee as to how your kids might react, however 'grown up' they're supposed to be. Despite being in their forties children can struggle to see their parents as independent adults, and even if they left home years before, they may still be traumatized by Mummy and Daddy splitting up. But life is hard and some things are quite shit.

For those of us who stick it out, most midlife relationships are a compromise and millions of us are cool with that. You annoy him, he gets on your tits, but if he's late home and the idea of him being dead in a ditch still upsets you, then hang on in there. (If, on the other hand, the idea of him being dead in a ditch becomes a bit of a fantasy, then it might be time to start talking to your lawyers.)

Whatever your circumstances in middle-age, whether you're blissfully/resentfully married, blissfully/resentfully single, dating, cohabiting, whatever, you will often find yourself being pulled in all sorts of directions, and shockingly, all of a sudden you are the one who is considered the grown-up, the one who's expected to solve all sorts of problems.

It can be very daunting realizing that you might have to take on some responsibility for your mum and dad, when up until now you've secretly harboured the thought that if the worse came to the worst, you could always run home to Mummy and Daddy and they'd kiss it all better. Now it's you who has to kiss everything better, and the problems you're faced with in midlife tend to be the big ones – the life-and-death ones, the ones you don't have any answers for, and certainly not the ones that can be kissed better. You are the 'responsible adult', the one who should know the name of the family solicitor and whether your parents want to be resuscitated, buried or cremated? Fortunately, I'm the middle child of three and my older sister went to law school, so I can still play thick when she's around, but for many of us, this is the time when we have to step up to the plate.

Because this is also when the family dog needs to be put down and your children start having grown-up problems of their own. Children are an emotional battlefield at any age, but once they can't be comforted by a small toy and/or some sweets, and they start wading into areas you can't control, that's when your real problems begin.

With women having babies later in life, many mothers find themselves menopausal at exactly the same time their children hit their teens. Oh great! Just when you could really do with a decent night's sleep, this is when they start staggering home from parties three hours after their curfew and, once again, you worry they might choke to death on their own sick in the night. This is when they need hoiking out of police stations and start accepting lifts from people who passed their driving test two days earlier and decide they've always hated playing the piano, even though they're naturally gifted and on the brink of getting Grade 8. Aaaaaaagh!

On top of that, you've still got a massive mortgage because once upon a time someone persuaded you that 'interest only' was a really good idea, plus there's a funny smell on the landing, a damp patch in the bedroom that's not in the right place (i.e. it's on the ceiling and not the bed) and the washing machine is making those really ominous death-rattle noises.

This is why the menopause is so difficult to deal with. For the majority, it arrives at the most inconvenient time of your life, when you are pathologically tired for no reason and your feet hurt, you really need your sleep and you simply don't have time to worry about anything else.

So the menopause has a habit of catching you out when you're at your most vulnerable. It tends to coincide with a time when even having fun starts to feel like hard work. Everything begins to take its toll. You can't so much as look at a lump of cheese without the top button flying off your trousers, suddenly a sip over three small glasses of wine and you wake up the next day feeling like someone ran you over in the night and, to top it all, your hormones go into some kind of biological meltdown and no amount of diary planning or being organized can help with random periods which either last for twenty minutes or have you sitting on the loo not daring to move for thirty-six hours in case you leave a bloodied trail around the neighbourhood. A bit like that film what's-his-name did. And that's another thing – you won't be able to remember anything: names, dates, PIN numbers . . . (Every PIN number you have will need to be written down on a tiny piece of paper and hidden in that secret compartment in your purse which, by the way, every bag snatcher and purse thief knows about.)

On top of all this, your husband/partner, if you've still got one, will be entertaining some kind of midlife crisis of their own and dismantling motorbikes on the sitting-room carpet or going vegan and buying a great deal of Lycra cycling gear.

What I'm trying to say is that, when the menopause hits, nothing feels normal any more and when you can't control your hormones it's very difficult to control anything else – be it your appetite, temper or tongue. Hence, as the squashed bit of manky ham in the generational sandwich, you will find yourself snapping and saying really vile things to your nearest and dearest and, consequently, rows escalate quicker than if someone chucked kerosene into the mix.

Then the entire atmosphere in the house will change. I swear I began to create a lot of static electricity around me and started experiencing a huge number of electric shocks. Getting in and out of my car was enough to create sparks. And as for the hand rail in

Peter Jones, just the briefest touch had me jumping about three feet in the air, whilst I have never been able to use a self-service till due to my temper static interfering with the bar-code reading.

So the menopause doesn't just affect you; it affects everyone around you. Your family might start hiding sharp knives, they will start walking on eggshells around you, will certainly discuss you behind your back and are most likely to agree that you are in the process of 'losing it' slightly. (This will be because you have neatly stashed the soap and shampoo in the fridge and the chilli sauce and mayonnaise in the bathroom cabinet; that said, mayonnaise is a great bathroom cabinet stand by, because when you've run out of everything else, it makes a mighty fine moisturizer.)

The thing to remember whilst you are riding this emotional bucking bronco is that all the chaos is normal. It's what millions of us are going through, every minute of every day. You're in good company.

And with this in mind, one of the plusses of the menopause is that I think it signals a time when women start to really sympathize with each other. The sisterhood becomes properly solid because right now we have a great deal in common. As a younger woman fighting hard for my career I wasn't as supportive of other women as I should have been because I was jealous of them. This jealousy was badly exacerbated by the nature of the business I was in. Back in the 1980s and 90s the world of women in comedy was very competitive: if one of us made it through the magic door into Successville, it often meant the door was swiftly slammed shut behind them for a good long while after. It seemed we were only let through that door one at a time and the idea of more than one woman ever appearing on a comedy quiz show or panel game was still a distant dream. There was very little equality in terms of balancing the sexes on screen and sadly, back then, when a fellow lady stand-up struck it lucky, I couldn't help feeling it would be at my expense: she had won, therefore I had lost. All that guff is over now. I have neither the time nor the inclination to be petty; there's room for everyone – we all just need to budge up a bit.

Menopausal women also have a great deal of shared experience, and I'm not just talking about the common physical side effects of the medical hoop we find ourselves jumping through. I'm talking about all the other life experiences that go hand in hand with being a certain age. By the time we hit the menopause, there are very few women who will not have experienced loss, who don't know what it is to grieve. All of us will have weathered our own private storms, battled our own demons and known our own crashing disappointments. I think this makes us nicer to each other. We recognize the struggle in each other's lives – we get it, we understand, we know what it's like to try and juggle everything and how it feels when we keep dropping the balls.

That's why it's our unspoken duty to step in and help when we see someone having a tough time, whether it's handing someone change for a public convenience or passing them a tissue when they're crying on the bus. The great thing about being older is that we're not embarrassed to hold out a hand.

PS On the subject of mums and dads here, if they're still alive when you hit fifty, you are really lucky. Cherish them and don't forget to ask them questions. They're not like us, they don't Instagram and blog, and they stopped taking photos years ago, so all their memories are in their heads. Ask them to share some of these before they die or forget them. Every time I see my mum, I want to ask her these things, but as soon as I walk into her flat we start bickering about whether you can hear a word Fiona Bruce says and how long broccoli takes to steam and the opportunity slips by yet again.

T

TIME

'In the old days, the menopause used to be called "the change of life" (so called because your life does change, and it all happens so fast: one minute you're snogging boys down back alleys, the next minute you don't like driving at night).' **JE**

There is nothing like the Big M to remind you that time is marching on. Bearing in mind the average age to begin the menopause is fifty-one, then, lady, mathematically, once those periods dry up, you are more than likely to be over halfway through your life.

Now despite middle age being a bit of a drag both physically and mentally, those of us who are going through it have got to appreciate that there are many women who never made it this far and that, sweaty sheets and brain fog aside, we are lucky to be here. We're also lucky to be living in an age when there is so much more awareness about the menopausal condition. Once upon a time, it was all rather taboo and women thought they might die of shame if they spoke openly about what they were experiencing, never mind approach their inevitably male doctors to discuss their symptoms. Women didn't even discuss how grim they were feeling with their own friends.

I always remember years ago, back in the 1970s, a fifty-something friend of my mother's completely lost it one Christmas Day and locked herself in the garage for the duration of the festivities. Looking back, it was such an obvious menopausal cry for help, but no one twigged at the time and it was all swept under the carpet never to be mentioned again.

Society has become much better at airing collective grubby laundry. Daytime TV is much maligned, but for many of us the topics relating to women's health that are discussed on programmes such as *Good Morning Britain* and *Loose Women* make us feel more normal about what we're experiencing. And this includes the menopause. Basically, if other people own up to going through the same thing, then it normalizes the situation: there's safety in numbers, girls! In fact, I think daytime TV is not only instrumental in making women feel better about their health problems, I think it can save lives. So well done, daytime telly – keep telling it like it is.

The people who really don't help the menopausal cause are those who are in complete denial; those who are skittish about their age and try to turn the clock back on their faces by having a ton of work done.

Listen, you can do what you like. I'm not anti-Botox. I've never had any, but sometimes I pull my chins up behind my ears and imagine what it would be like to have a nice, neat jawline again. So I don't blame women for having the bags removed from their eyes or massive noses trimmed. However, the truth is that you can nip and tuck as much as you like, but inside, your internal organs are going off at the same rate as everyone else's. You may not look as menopausal as the rest of us, but you'll feel it. And anyway, the under-arm sweat rings are a dead hot-flush giveaway – unless, of course, you have had your sweat glands Botoxed too. (**Fact:** if you do suffer from excessive sweating, then Botox can be the answer and a good dermatologist should be able to advise. Apparently, all the big-name actresses have it done before a red-carpet event, in case, God forbid, they are seen to perspire. Honestly, one day I'd like to see a fifty-something actress with a great big grey middle parting, shuffling down a red carpet in a pair of slippers, exposing unshaven legs through a dressing gown – but then I'm just a cynical old biddy.)

CHANGES AND CHOICES

Although the phrase 'the change of life' might have fallen out of fashion, the sentiment could be more useful than you'd imagine. Let's face it: your life *has* changed and it's no good pretending that it hasn't. So maybe this is the time to start taking real stock of the situation you are in and make any changes to the way you're living before it really is too late. And when I say this, I'm not talking about downsizing and moving to the country/France/Timbuktu. Those are massive decisions that I couldn't possibly advise you on. (That said, I think moving to the country is far harder than people expect; ideally, when I'm a little old lady I'd like to live within staggering distance of Tate Britain, sod the duck pond.)

But back to the point. I'm talking about eliminating anything you really don't like, whether that means culling a pile of coats in the hallway that no one has worn for years or giving up on a book you're just not enjoying. Because life really is too short. In fact, life is too short for many things.

LIFE IS TOO SHORT . . .

- Life is too short to spend time with people who make you feel crap. You might have known them for years, but

---

it doesn't matter – if they drain the life blood out of you, drop 'em. (**PS** They probably don't like you much either.)

- Life is too short to sit through the second half of a dreadful play. Remember, intervals aren't just for getting drinks and having a wee, you know. If you're bored out of your skull, this is your chance to escape.

- Life is too short to eat a lousy meal in an expensive restaurant. Complain loudly and leave; there's usually a Nando's not far away.

- Life is too short to be angry with someone without telling them why. I'm a firm believer that sulking and bottling it up is very bad for your health. Let it all out before it poisons you from the inside.

- Life is too short not to say sorry. Once you get into the habit of saying sorry, it gets easier and it's incredible how much better it can make you feel. Obviously, occasionally, you may not actually *be* sorry, but hopefully it'll sound convincing enough to clear the air.

- Life is too short not to try something new, even if it's just a different type of pickle (if in doubt, put it on the side of your plate rather than smearing it all over your food; I learned this the hard way when it came to kimchi).

- Life is too short not to stuff a mushroom, if you enjoy stuffing mushrooms – or other veg (peppers, tomatoes, aubergines, etc.). Stuff what you like.

- Life is too short to hate your hair without attempting to do something about it. Ditto weight, however . . .

- . . . life is also too short to keep that pair of shorts you're never going to squeeze your arse back into. Chuck 'em.

Now is the time to take control of the day-to-day and attempt to make even the boring stuff more enjoyable. For example, tackling a huge mound of ironing is far less dreary when you've got a brilliant audio book on the go, *fact*.

Basically, the menopause was a bit of a watershed for me, and my life has definitely divided into before and after. Yes, there are things I miss about the physically younger me, and sometimes looking at photos of me when I was in my thirties and even forties can be a bit painful. But mentally, I prefer the me I am now. I've got a much better grip on who I am and what I *want* versus what I *need*: I *want* more money, better clothes, more exotic holidays; do I *need* them? No.

ME TIME

As I've got older, I've decided to take more time doing the things I like, whether that's my hobbies or spending longer on the phone with my mum. I've also decided to take the time to do things the way I like them. For example, I like my coffee made with hot milk – it only takes thirty seconds to heat the milk up in the microwave and it makes all the difference.

I've spent so much of my life rushing things, I never realized how much better everything is if you just slow down a bit and savour the moment. These days, I really am taking time to smell the roses, I'm picking my fruit more carefully in the supermarket and checking to see if those avocados are ripe enough (I'm even trying to drink wine slower).

I've always kind of sneered at the phrase 'me time', but finally

I'm beginning to get it. Although one woman's me time is another woman's bore time (personally, I don't want to sit around having my nails painted drinking Prosecco – I loathe Prosecco – but I understand for some women this is a precious treat).

My 'me time' includes stopping work on writing days at 7pm to listen to *The Archers*. It's simple and it's free, but it always feels like a bit of a reward, as I lie on the bed, wiggle my toes and let other people's fictional lives wash over me. Other 'me time' favourites include *Antiques Roadshow, Masterchef, Bake Off* and *Sewing Bee*. Television is a much-maligned art form. At its best, it's something that can unite the nation; at its worst, it's *The Masked Singer*, which is still brilliant.

TECHNOLOGY AND TIME

Time goes faster the older you get and the menopause is a great big warning that from now on things are only going to speed up. These days, Christmas seems to roll around every six months and birthdays are just as bad – before you know it you're sixty, then seventy, then eighty, then ninety . . .

We're lucky to be ageing in the twenty-first century with technology on our side. In the old days, if we suddenly felt the need to get in touch with an old mate, we'd have to start by tracking down an address and then messing about with paper, pen and a stamp. Now the Internet can hook us up in moments. Thanks to email, social media and texts, keeping in touch with people is so much easier and cheaper than it ever used to be. It's up to us to take advantage of this.

I know that social media is often frowned upon, but used by us grown-ups it can be an incredible comfort. Thanks to Twitter, I've got an army of similarly aged women on whom I feel I can rely for laughs/ sympathy/news/gossip. If you haven't tried it, I'd suggest you have a go. For starters, there are plenty of Twitter menopause groups out there – some professional, others more of a friendly support network. Believe me, if you have a menopausal medical problem or query, someone on Twitter will have an answer. Though as ever: if in doubt, see your doctor.

Instagram is also rather good fun, if you like gawping at pictures of other people's lives, though this can prove unhealthy if, like me, you're the jealous type.

A healthier way, possibly, to spend your time is to use technology to learn something new. I could lose hours to YouTube painting tutorials, for example. Have a gander: they cover all levels and media and might be just the thing to get you going.

We are the first generation of menopausal women to have all the knowledge in the world under our own roofs. Technology is our friend. It's good to keep up with it because, as we get older, it's going to get more and more useful. I recently bought my ninety-year-old mother June an Alexa, so that she could ask her simple time, date and weather questions (my mother's sight is not what it was and she misses her newspapers). She is unfailingly polite to this bit of techno kit, but recently insisted it was broken. Hmmmm . . . No, it wasn't. My mum just couldn't remember her name and Alexa simply wasn't going to respond to being called Alison, Annie or Imogen.

CALLING TIME ON THE MENOPAUSE

In the summer of 2019, the *Sunday Times* broke a story about a new medical procedure called 'ovarian tissue cryopreservation' which a private clinic in Birmingham had already begun offering to women up to the age of forty.

Also known as 'ovarian grafting', the procedure can delay the menopause by up to twenty years, meaning that rather than experiencing the menopause in your fifties, you could be in your seventies, hot flushing it through the bridge and bingo.

By all accounts, the keyhole surgery takes around thirty minutes, is relatively painless and involves taking a piece of ovarian tissue which is then deep frozen, ready to be thawed out and re-grafted once the woman approaches her menopause. The re-grafted tissue then kick-starts the ovaries into thinking they are young again and, hey presto, for around £11K, you can be menopause free for up to two decades.

Ok, this is brilliant news for young women who, through cancer treatment and other devastating fertility issues (including hysterectomies due to endometriosis), are facing hormonal freefall into an early menopause years before they otherwise would. Instead of dealing with more medical misery, these women will be spared feeling both physically and psychologically prematurely middle-aged, which seems pretty fair to me. It could also be a miracle cure for those who have a family history of early menopause and for whom the op might be an insurance against running out of time to have children.

I have sympathy with all these women and I hope the treatment soon becomes available for those who really need it on the NHS. What bothers me, however, is that because this treatment is available to all women under forty who can afford it, we might be looking at a future where the rich are no longer bothering with all that messy menopause nonsense and choosing to live night-sweat and brain-fog free, unlike the rest of us plebs who will be sweating it out, eating biscuits and searching desperately for the libido we seem to have lost down the back of the sofa.

And there is also another issue here of women continuing to be fertile into their late sixties. Imagine accidentally getting up the duff just before your seventieth.

But maybe I'm just jealous because this revolutionary new treatment has come too late to be any good to me. Hmmm . . . possibly? Here's an extract from an article I wrote for the *Independent* the week the news broke, which I think sums up my feelings:

I suppose the thing that bothers me most is that there's an element to this that smacks of the usual distaste for women getting older. How dare we be hot and sweaty and go round slamming doors? Wouldn't it be better all round if women just signed up for a tiny bit of keyhole surgery and went about their business in a cuter and more sexy way until they die?

Please don't think for a moment I'm dismissing the incredible life changing difference this pioneering treatment can do for the people who need it, especially if it restores fertility to women who would like to have children, how miraculous is that?

I have a problem dealing with the concept that because the menopause is considered unattractive, we should do away with it, or put it off until you're really old and ugly because who cares how you cope with it then? At least you won't be at work, huffing around the office, annoying everyone by opening every window and crying over leaving your favourite scarf on the bus.

I find the idea of having to deal with the menopause on top of every other geriatric health problem slightly off-putting. Imagine changing the batteries in your hearing aid whilst having a hot flush. No thanks.

For me, the menopause has been a rite of passage and yes, parts of it have been uncomfortable and annoying, but it has also been interesting. It has changed me as a person and it has made me so much more aware of who I really am.

But then a lot of people would argue that as I don't have a proper job, I wouldn't really know what it's like to be menopausal in the workplace, to which I say: it's 2019, the workplace is dealing with vast numbers of people, all of whom have all types of problems; we are better at this kind of stuff than we used to be, we're better at being kinder to people who are struggling with all sorts of things from period pains to eating disorders and anxiety. Let's not turn the empathy clock back.

Of course, all women deal with their menopause differently. Personally, after some spectacular slanging matches on the street, I went down the HRT route to help with my anger issues; others choose to bite down hard on leather. What I don't think we should do though, is turn this into a condition to be avoided at all costs.

There's a great deal about being a middle-aged menopausal woman that is a bit of a drag. The weight thing I could do without, but then I could do without eating great big slabs of cheese. However, there's a great deal to celebrate too and as I approach sixty, thanks to the menopause, I am better at being me than I ever have been.

U

UNUSUAL SYMPTOMS

'I met a middle-aged air hostess recently who told me that, whilst she might not be the youngest or fittest of the cabin crew, she's the only one who can fart the entire length of a jumbo jet, from steerage through business and first class, all the way to the cockpit. With age comes wisdom . . . and wind.' **JE**

There is no such thing as a textbook menopause, no two women will experience exactly the same symptoms for exactly the same length of time, and quite frankly, some of the side effects that some of us ladies suffer from can be pretty weird.

Like the above-mentioned air hostess, I find that some days I let off almost constantly. The other day, I was taking the laundry upstairs and I farted on every step (well, actually, I missed one out, so I went back for it!).

But excessive trumping is not the only peculiar symptom in this process. This chapter features a selection of surprising menopausal conditions, both physical and psychological that will a) either help you to identify something that's been bothering you for a while, or b) make you think, Well at least I haven't got *that*!

POP-SOCK LEG

A debilitating condition, which can prove fatal if the pop sock is not removed quickly enough. It's basically caused by purchasing an over-tight pop sock and encasing a fat calf within. As the day progresses, and your legs swell because you're on your feet and it's hot, the welt of the pop sock will start to form an indentation around the flesh under the knee. Should this welt turn purple, you are in danger of cutting off your supply of oxygen to the brain and the pop sock must be removed before confusion sets in. Let this be a warning to you.

LAKELANDITIS

One of the most peculiar symptoms of the menopause is that, despite having spent most of your life being a domestic slut, you find that as your oestrogen levels drop, your interest in household products increases. Most commonly, this will manifest itself in hours spent browsing the Lakeland catalogue, wondering whether to treat your-self to a new cutlery tidy or an adjustable chopping board storage rack?

There is something so delightful about the world of Lakeland that I don't know why they don't turn it into a theme park for middle-aged women, complete with rides featuring giant rolling pins, swinging gravy boats and merry-go-rounds in the shape of salad spinners. It would be even better than Legoland. Overheating matrons would be encouraged to take off all their clothes and run naked through the 'Garden Sprinkler Experience' – a kind of bracing cold car wash for the menopausal. Or, for the less adventurous, there would be a life-size gingerbread house to explore.

Whilst we wait for this to happen, you can always visit a shop. Lakeland is the Ann Summers for the fifty-something female. Because, let's face it, at our age most of us can bring ourselves to orgasm at the prospect of a really well-ordered laundry area.

TEMPER STATIC

Not all menopausal women will experience temper static, but those who do – like me – will find that it can seriously impact everyday life.

Temper static is triggered by getting hysterical in a frustrating situation. For example, trying to use a parking app that refuses to recognize your car number plate or attempting to scan your items at a self-service till in the supermarket. This is something I have yet to successfully achieve because, thanks to 'temper static', I have some spooky Carrie-like inability to scan my items. Which means I'm a nightmare in a busy supermarket in rush hour and people think I'm mucking about on purpose, but I promise I'm not. The problem lies in the fact that once my temper levels have been raised, the resulting electrical static interferes with the analogue signal generated by the reflected light required to decode the digits on my item and my bar codes refuse to scan. And it doesn't seem to matter how I present my goods, where I stand or at what distance. Seriously, I've tried every which way.

Say I've got a tub of coleslaw (I call it crack cabbage; let's just say I've got a bit of a habit), I might start the process by casually waving the item under the little red light, ever so nonchalantly as if to catch it off guard. When that doesn't work, I usually resort to shaking the thing aggressively, muttering, 'Come on you thick twat, just work you fucking imbecile.' At other times, when I'm not in a hurry, I will proffer my shopping like a sugar cube under the nose of a shy pony, ever so gently like a fully trained till whisperer: 'Look, see, you know what this is don't you, so why don't you make that nice beeping noise for Mummy?' But no, nine times out of ten I have to call for an assistant and explain, through my tears, that 'I caaaan't do it', whereupon, because they're young and don't exude temper static from every pore, they proceed to whisk my items into the bagging area, like a magician, whilst I stand back in awe.

DESICCATION

The inability to retain any moisture whatsoever during the menopause is kind of crazy. In the past I've described the process as turning into a pterodactyl from the neck down – because boy, have I got scaly. Podcast Judith once said that every time she took her tights off there was a blizzard of shin dandruff and she's not alone. I've always been a dry-skinned woman but mid-menopause I realized that there wasn't any bit of my body that hadn't dried out (see also Chapter V for Vaginas). In fact, I realized I had so much dry, cracked skin on my heels that if I had it all removed, I'd be a good three inches shorter.

Hand in hand with the dry skin, came the itchy red rash which flared up around my neck whenever I wore my favourite (and very expensive) perfume. In despair, I went to see a dermatologist and was diagnosed with eczema. Grrrrrrr. Since then, I've had to forgo my daily treat of a heavily scented bath and these days the only thing I'm allowed in the tub with me are unperfumed soaps and a liquid-paraffin preparation which comes in a huge, ugly plastic dispenser which basically screams 'problem skin'.

Oh yes, and at the age of fifty-seven I developed a wart on my forehead. Proof, if ever it were needed, that there is a bit of witch in all menopausal women. However, as my mother pointed out: 'At least it's not on the end of your nose, haha.' (But I had it frozen off anyway, because growing my fringe long enough to cover it meant that I kept bumping into lamp posts.)

On a more serious note about the whole drying-up process, the most shocking and upsetting thing I developed as a menopausal woman was dry-eye syndrome, which basically does what it says in the title: your eyes dry up and, left untreated, they feel itchy and uncomfortable. Even watching television can be tricky without using drops, whilst reading small print becomes downright impossible. This is one of those harmless, 'it-won't-kill-you' conditions, but it is chronic (as in once you've got it, it won't go away) and, to be honest, it's a complete drag. According to the experts on Google, dry eye is very common amongst the ageing population, and whilst men do get it, the majority of sufferers are female. And . . . guess what? It often begins as a result of hormonal changes. Oh, here we go again, girls!

I had a massive panic attack when I was first diagnosed with dry eye. Knowing it wasn't going to magically get better really upset me and I spiralled into a state of advanced anxiety causing my mouth to dry out. A quick Google of both dry eye and dry mouth led me to believe I'd developed a debilitating disease called Sjögren's syndrome, which the tennis player Venus Williams has been dealing with for a number of years. Sjögren's can be a nightmare both to diagnose and treat. In the end, I was sent for tests at King's College Hospital in London which has a specialist Sjögren's clinic where I was eventually persuaded that I didn't have the condition. However, despite conclusive evidence that I wasn't a Sjögren's sufferer, my mental state remained very off balance and I had what my mother refers to as a 'teeny nervous breakdown'. Talking therapy was advised (AKA seeing a shrink) and I had a go, but the woman annoyed me. Eventually, I fell under the spell of an incredible acupuncturist who lives around the corner and has healing in her hands (and needles).

Several years on from the dry-eye diagnosis, it's still a huge daily bore but I manage it. I type in a twenty-point font so as not to strain my eyes, sleep in a room with a humidifier, apply microwaved hot masks (available online), use the drops as often as I need to and at night I sleep with cling film patches over my eyes. This is the detail that always freaks everyone out and, yes, it is weird, but I was given the tip at Moorfields Eye Hospital, and if it's good enough for them . . . Anyway, here's what I do: every single night, without fail, I fill my eyes up with an over-the-counter ointment which is sold specifically for night-time dry-eye treatment (I use VitA-POS but other brands are also available). Once my eyes are completely gummed up with this runny Vaseline-like substance, I cut two two-inch squares from a roll of cling film (which I keep under the bed) and plaster one over each eye. Weirdly, the cling film sticks to the skin and, despite moving around quite a bit, the patches don't come adrift in the night. The cling film works because it provides a moisture chamber for the eyes, the ointment soaks in gradually overnight moisturizing the eyeballs and for a few hours in the morning, until about midday, I don't need drops or anything. In fact, until then, my eyes feel pretty normal.

As for the day-time, artificial tear drops are the way to go. Visit any pharmacy and you will be faced with a mind-boggling choice of dry-eye drops. Sadly, it's trial and error as to which will work best for you and it can be an expensive process. My golden rule is to search for anything that does *not* contain preservatives because, as I found out to my cost, these can make the problem a great deal worse.

For those who can afford it, there are a growing number of dry-eye clinics in the bigger cities across the country, so if you're really suffering, it might a good idea to pop into one of these and see if you're a suitable candidate for a procedure which certainly helped me. I had LipiFlow at Optical Express in Shaftesbury Avenue, London – a totally painless treatment that gave me nine months of relief. Sadly, it's expensive (around £800 for both eyes) and, despite being effective, it's not a cure. However, I'm saving up for another go, as I've heard the more you have it done, the longer it lasts. That said, they will only treat you once in any twelve-month period. There are other dry-eye treatments available, but considering this was my personal experience I thought I should share it in the hope that it might help you or someone you know.

PS If you do go down the cling-film route and spend as much time in hotels as I do, always make sure you've put the roll back in your suitcase before going down for breakfast. I've lost track of the number of times my cling film has been discovered under the bed by a chambermaid who must wonder what kind of kinky sex games I get up to on my own in a Travellodge. Now that's what I call rock 'n' roll.

VAGINAS

'There are many names for the vagina. Mine's called Elaine.' **JE**

The vagina, as anyone who has ever witnessed a woman giving birth will know, is an incredible and weirdly flexible part of our anatomy – as stretchy as a gymnast, its construction is quite complicated, as you'll also know if you've ever attempted to get down there with a mirror. (By the way, this can be quite a tricky procedure, especially if you're short sighted, but . . . hold on . . . I've finally realized the one good use for a selfie stick! Because, if you think about it, a selfie stick is the ideal instrument with which to view your noo. You could even take a close-up for posterity; although I'd advise against putting it up on Instagram – you might just lose a few followers.)

The trouble with getting a proper look at your love tunnel is that unless you're a contortionist with 20/20 vision, it's a bit of a jumble of folds and holes and if you have a great deal of pubic hair, then it's a bit like trying to find a rabbit warren in an overgrown forest.

For years I was really confused about where the wee-wee hole was in relation to the actual opening of the vagina. (For those still in doubt, they're pretty close, with the urethral opening sitting neatly just below the clitoris.)

If it's been years since you've seen a vagina, either your own or anyone else's, it's easy to have an online Google check, just to remind yourself of quite how clever and mad it is.

For starters, the vagina is unbelievably multi-functional, what with it being the go-to area for sex, birth and menstruation. Hence our relationship with it can become a bit love/hate. (Maybe men would have a completely different relationship with their sex organs if their penises bled heavily for a week once a month!)

But as this is a book about the menopause, at this stage we can safely guess that for you, dear reader, the periods are over (or on their way out) and the vagina should be sitting happily in one's big cotton knickers, occasionally being called on for rumpy-pumpy duties. By the way, I state cotton knickers here, because anyone wearing a nylon gusset at any age is just asking for trouble – or 'thrush', as it's medically known.

Obviously, there are many things that can go wrong with the fanny, and it's very important that you attend your smear tests, even if you are no longer sexually active. It's also vital to see your GP if something's bothering you, especially if that 'something' can't be solved with over-the-counter medications. Let's not forget, there are five gynae cancers and awareness of symptoms is proven to be lower than it should be. So don't ignore anything that triggers an alarm bell; your GP is better placed than you (or the Internet) to decide if things need further investigation.

Sadly, as many of us will have experienced, the vagina, being the intricate piece of kit that it is, doesn't age particularly well. Like an old car that's gone a bit rusty in the garage and occasionally needs its bonnet popping in order to give it some oil, the vagina's biggest problem is dryness.

LOTIONS AND LUBE

Ok, so let's just talk properly about vaginal dryness here. I understand it's probably different for everyone, but when I first developed it, it wasn't what I was expecting at all. I thought vaginal dryness would be a very general thing, a bit like having dandruff. I thought the entire vulval area would look and feel a bit raw and that the actual inside of the vagina would no longer feel wet. What I wasn't expecting was the very deep itch that came from one specific spot – for me, it's at the bottom of the vulva, on the left-hand side, quite near the perineum – and lord, when it's having a bad day it's like a thousand ants burrowing down one nerve ending and the urge to claw at the area is almost irresistible. In my case, over-the-counter remedies work up to a point, but every few months I find myself at the doctor's begging for a short course of something a bit more heavy duty and she will prescribe me a steroid cream just to really calm things down.

I have never suffered with an internally dry foo – my vaginal canal is still pretty juicy – but for millions of women this is the thing that causes the greatest discomfort when attempting sex. In which case, yours is the basket with the lube in, lady, and there is no shame in using it.

When we are young, the vagina keeps its tissues soft and moist thanks to the glands near the cervix producing slightly acidic moisture which moves down the vagina, preventing infection and removing dead skin cells. (This appeared as that white discharge in our gussets which we used to worry about, thinking it might mean we were dirty, when in actual fact it was a sign that everything was completely tickety-boo.)

During sexual excitement more moisture is produced by the two Bartholin's glands, which are near the entrance to the vagina, and this natural lubrication prevents friction during sex. Clever stuff, but obviously as we get older, these glands start to malfunction and we need some help in the moisture department.

Now the variety of lubrication on offer is quite mind-boggling and, speaking as someone who has developed stupidly sensitive skin as I've got older, to the point where I've been warned against using soaps containing parabens (non-scented chemical preservatives) which, coincidentally, are also found in some lubricants, I'd recommend that you do your homework. The last thing you need is something that sets your fanny on fire in completely the wrong way. And don't, whatever you do, buy anything scented, coloured or, God help us, with glitter in it. Why anyone would want to have the vaginal secretions of a My Little Pony is completely beyond me, but it's available!

THE VAGISAN AD

When I was fifty-eight and, weirdly, had just been diagnosed as having vaginal dryness (which, to be honest, was a relief, as I was convinced it was something a great deal more sinister), I got one of those telephone calls from my management which begin with the words, 'Er . . . not sure how you're going to feel about this, but . . . We've had this offer . . . '

The offer in question was for me to front a TV campaign for a well-known and respected brand of vaginal moisturizing cream. The company (Dr Wolff), who are German and had been in the business for many years, believed passionately in their product, which quite simply is an over-the-counter hormone-free cream which can be applied to the vagina by hand (finger) or via a plastic applicator, for those who are more squeamish about such things.

I must admit, I did have a good, long think about it. I knew there would be some social-media snideness – it was inevitable – so I discussed it with my family, none of whom seemed remotely bothered by the prospect.

The fee was generous, I had script approval, I liked the set and they bought me a nice new shirt and a lovely pair of bright pink suede loafers, which I still refer to as my Vagisan shoes.

What I hadn't accounted for was how often the ad would be repeated and the fact that it seemed to be on at peak viewing times. Now this didn't bother me – it showed the company had faith in the ad and were happy to pay for the top slots. However, it did bother quite a lot of other people, mostly fathers of young families who were infuriated that their family viewing should be interrupted by such obscenity – apparently, their kids were asking questions! This, of course, was all my fault: it was unnecessary and embarrassing. Sometimes I'd try to appease these Twitter haters, telling them that children really didn't care much about anything as long as they were given a straight answer; a simple 'it's a problem old ladies get' would do. But sometimes I'd get fed up and threaten that next time I'd demonstrate the product with my knickers off.

I understand some families have a pretty low blush threshold, but I do think that reacting to a pretty innocuous ad with howls of disgust in front of children is setting up problems for the future: hmm, so bodily functions are disgusting, are they? Better not tell Dad I've started my periods. And so the circle of shame begins.

I also got a bit of grief from women, which was depressing, because I always assume we're better off having each other's backs rather than calling each other out for being 'gross'. I was also pretty devastated by some comments from the gay fraternity, a few of whom felt the need to tell me how 'icky' it was. There were also quite a number of accusations of having lost whatever career I'd ever had. Hmmmm . . . I don't think so. In fact, I'm really proud of that job. Not just because I am the first person to have said 'vaginal dryness' during a TV ad in this country, but also because it's only thanks to advertising Vagisan moisture cream that I have any pension whatsoever. Cheers, Dr Wolff.

FEMALE-PATTERN BALDING

Back in 2005, Podcast Judith and I met up to write the first in a series of *Grumpy Old Women Live* shows. Judith had been the producer on the highly successful *Grumpy Old Women* TV series, and I'd been one of the regular contributors. That first *Live* show was a career highlight: it went on tour and sold out all over the country, before touring Australia and being translated into Finnish and Icelandic.

One of the great things about doing the show was realizing how universal a great deal of women's comedy is, particularly when it gets down to the nitty gritty of ageing. There was a joke in that show which referred to 'female-pattern balding' – a euphemism for the thinning of one's pubes. All these years on, I still remember the punchline, which went: 'Of course, the real problem with female-pattern balding is whether to shave it all off or comb it over.' Cue, BIG LAUGH.

The fact that this joke worked even when it was translated into other languages was a testament to how much menopausal women around the world have in common, which is strangely comforting.

WARDROBLE DILEMMAS

'I've seen salads that are better dressed than me. I don't even know where to buy my clothes from any more – if I go into Top Shop, everyone thinks I'm the store detective.' **JE**

Having once been a woman who strode around the stage in a pair of size ten red PVC trousers, realizing that I have spent most of the past decade wearing trousers with elasticated waists could be seen as depressing. But what would be even more depressing would be squashing myself into a pair of size fourteen/sixteen red PVC trousers and looking like something that fell off the back of a cheap sofa delivery van.

Of course, what I really need is a good dose of dysentery to kick-start a diet and fitness regime, but sadly, I have a cast-iron stomach, and despite prising open mussels, buying kebabs from disgusting late-night joints and never wiping down my raw-meat board, nothing has ever give me even the mildest of squits. It's really not fair.

I didn't expect to be this tubby little creature in my fifties. I thought I was going to grow up to be one of those rather elegant, Levis/white shirt/loafer-wearing women, only with a slightly edgy rock-chick twist – a sort of cross between Patti Smith and Debbie Harry. Oh, but no. Somehow, over the years, I've morphed into one of those Shreddies knitting nanas and sometimes, if I'm not careful, I can end up being very lazy about making an effort to dress nicely.

I think a lot of us stop making an effort to dress up when we're menopausal because we can't see the point. It's that vicious circle of I-feel-fat-therefore-I-might-as-well-look-like-a-frump. When in actual fact, if you look around, stylish people come in all shapes and sizes and some of the most stylish are big girls. Now I'm not advocating snacking your way through the menopause – let's try and keep things a bit healthy here – but the fact is there is something about your hormones going haywire that results in a bit of extra padding, and that means having to tweak your clothing to accommodate your new shape.

For some women, it's the boobs that go mad and start straining like leashed puppies at the seams of their bras; for others, it's a bit of all-over extra blubber. But for the vast majority of us, it's the sudden appearance of the spare tyre that sends us into a wardrobe tailspin.

My spare tyre is like a child's rubber ring – it's designed not to slip off easily. Therefore, I've had to incorporate it into my fashion choices. The worst thing a woman can do when she's feeling emotionally fragile is to try and dress like she did in her skinny thirties. Wouldn't it be great if we could just accept the change and embrace the bulge, rather than feel ashamed for simply going up a size (or two).

It would also help if clothing manufacturers were a little more sympathetic to our needs. For starters, a little bit of re-labelling would do us all a favour:

- A size 8 should be a 'smug'.
- Size 10 – 'It won't last'.
- 12 – 'Nice one, well done'.

- 14 – 'Normal'.
- 16 – 'Juicy'.
- 18 – 'Curvilicious'.
- 20 – 'Big and bouncy'.
- 22 – 'Chunky'.

By the time you are fifty-odd, you should have come to terms with your body shape. For example, I'm a box and Podcast Judith is more of a pelican (thin legs, big chest), whereas, most annoyingly, my older sister is still shaped like a young girl (she's the one sporting trousers from the 1980s and a swimming costume which she wore diving off the top board at a girl guides swimming gala half a century ago).

My sister is one of those women who actually likes exercise, she goes kayaking for fun and would rather walk to the supermarket than drive. She does more steps every day than anyone who hasn't got a dog has any right to do and this is probably why she weighs 8 stone and wears knickers with a ladybird label. My sister could be a sixty-something fashion plate, but fortunately for me, she's not that interested and tends to spend most of her clothes budget on walking waterproofs and sportswear. Which reminds me, she is the only woman I know to look like a burned match in her wetsuit on a beach.

Thin women have their own fashion dilemmas, I suppose, but I just can't think what they are? Us chubsters, on the other hand . . . where do I start? What most middle-aged women need to get through these difficult years are tops that don't ride up and bottoms that don't cling. I think most of us would be prepared to pay a couple more quid for a few extra inches of fabric. One of my pet hates are tops that stop bang on the midriff and expose great mounds of wobbly white flesh whenever I lift up my arms. NO! Give me the same top that falls to the hip and covers my tummy whatever moves I make and I might buy it. In fact, I might buy it in several different colours.

Another thing we don't want is silly fads. So quit the cut-out shoulder nonsense, the beads and the fringing and give us well-cut garments in quality fabrics (no sweaty nylon, cheers) with sleeves and pockets. Always pockets.

God knows, I love clothes, but I'm no fashion guru. I also realize that for many middle-aged women splashing out on expensive items is a complete no-no. However, the likelihood is that, unless you're prepared to go out wrapped in your duvet (which at least fits), you will need a few new things. Which doesn't mean to say they need to be new-new. I have rarely ever bought a brand-new coat – vintage and charity shops are great for coat bargains; a few years ago, I picked up a fabulous fake leopard-skin number in a second-hand shop locally and only the tatty lining gave its heritage away. Fortunately, my local dry cleaner offers a brilliant repair service, and for a few extra quid I had the grubby old lining replaced with a fabulous peacock green silk.

Whilst we might have trouble buying clothes that look great and fit nicely, finding accessories that fit is a lot less traumatic. After all, no one has a head that is too fat for a hat. This is why middle-aged women are suckers for those little extras – bags, shoes and statement necklaces. Personally, I'm a fan of those massive scarves that draw attention away from the tummy bulge. If I could get away with a turban as well, that would be great. However, as a woman who already has to wear glasses, I have to be careful not to over-accessorize. Sadly, one cannot wear flamboyant glasses, earrings and a necklace all together – not unless you want to look like a) a Christmas tree or b) Su Pollard (which can be an occupational hazard if, like me, you have looked like Su Pollard's slightly dowdier long-lost twin for years).

The other fashion faux pas that us ladies of a certain age (and Podcast Judith in particular) find difficult to resist is the crime of 'over-matching'. It can be very tempting, for example, to team a teal-coloured jumper with teal-coloured tights and a teal-coloured scarf *and* a teal-coloured bag. Don't do this. Also, beware of overdoing the leopard skin: treat leopard skin like sherry – tiny doses work best. Sometimes when Judith comes into the podcast studio wearing an over-matching ensemble I have to confiscate one or two items and give her a strict reminder about the over-matching rule.

THE IMPORTANCE OF CARDIGANS

Whatever your weight and shape, your best friend throughout the menopause will be your cardigan. Cardigans are wasted on any other age group. No one needs a cardi like we do – in fact, the menopause should also be referred to as, 'the cardi time of life' because at no other time are we dealing with such extreme swings in temperature. Basically, as soon as you put your cardi on, you have to take it off: cardi on, cardi off, cardi inside out and back to front . . . And the biggest problem with cardi shedding is that it's very easy to mislay your cardi. I remember going utterly berserk when I thought I'd lost my grey cashmere cardi and spending a good twenty minutes running around the house trying to find it, screaming and crying, before realizing I'd tied it securely around my waist.

CANNY CARDI TIPS

It's really easy to customize a cheap old cardi with some interesting buttons. I once ripped off a Paul Smith design by snipping off the regular grey buttons on a grey cardi and replacing them with a variety of different pink substitutes, all of which I sewed on à la Paul Smith in a contrasting thread. I know – get me! (The fact that some of the substitute buttons didn't actually fit through the buttonholes is beside the point. No self-respecting menopausal woman ever does a cardi up anyway.)

There's nothing more depressing than splashing out on something expensive like a cashmere cardi, only to find six months later that it's been ravaged by moths. Here's a handy hint from my friend Suzie Blake who wittily hand-darns her moth holes with delicately embroidered silk moths, which I think is either meta or a bit satirical. Of course, there's an element of skill involved in this and I'd practise your embroidered moths on an old sock first.

The cardi-around-the-waist look is another middle-aged female wardrobe trick. The great thing about this look is that the cardi covers your arse and no one can really tell how much of your backside is arse and how much is cardi. Top tip, girls.

I love my cardigans so much they all have individual names, there's big yellow, little orange, sensible navy, easy black, chunky grey and TK Maxx pink. Then there's 'itchy grey', 'grey that fell out of the car', 'mismatched buttons' and 'half-price skyblue'. Ok, now I can feel you rolling your eyes, so I'll stop (oh, let's not forget 'darling mustard').

CLOTHES TO AVOID

For most women suffering from hot flushes, certain clothes suddenly become the enemy. For example, beware the polyester blouse: I once nearly set fire to the sofa when struggling with my Netflix buffering whilst wearing something containing a nylon mix.

Polo-neck jumpers are also an absolute no-no and, personally, I can't even look at an Aran jumper without wanting to strip off and stand under a cold shower. (Depressingly, I once told a young girl about my Aran phobia, but it fell on deaf ears – she didn't even know what an Aran jumper was. I blame the grandmothers; they're too busy going to zumba classes these days to knit complicated cable-knit sweaters in really thick cream-coloured wool.)

TROUSERS

Before you embark on a trouser-buying quest, make sure you are carrying plenty of snacks and headache pills – it's probably going to be a long day. Oh, and tissues too, as it's more than likely there will be tears in the changing room.

Finding trousers that fit is the bane of my life. For one thing, I need to tackle trouser-buying on a day when self-esteem is high, so that I can blame any disasters on the cut of the trousers rather than the shape of my body.

After years of trouser hell I, like so many other women before me, have succumbed to the go-to choice of the middle-aged woman. That's right: elasticated-waist/pull-ups that Marks and Spencer have been discreetly selling for years. They are advertised as a 'no-fuss option' for any 'smart casual occasion'. Basically, they have an elasticated waist, no zips and come in three lengths: short, regular and long. Dear reader, I'm a size fourteen 'short', which is why I am buying these trousers in the first place. Conveniently, they also wash and dry in the machine, and although they're never going to set the world on fire, you can dress them up, dress them down and, even more importantly, lounge around in them without any nasty zips digging in. Basically, they are the ultimate, 'Fat Lazy Girl's pull-up trousers', and if only they would advertise them as such on a great big sign in the shop – preferably with an arrow pointing to the exact rail – I might be able to find them without ferreting through loads of other black trousers first.

For anyone wanting to buy these, the model number on the waistband is T59/6293W and they cost £25 at the time of writing.

SHOES

Listen, we've got enough on our plates without heels. Heels are a waste of time. Some women wear them because they are under the delusion that if you lift fat four inches off the ground, it ceases to exist. It doesn't, it's just in greater danger of toppling over. If heels really made you look thinner, then every portly middle-aged man bulging out of his suit would adopt them. But the fact is, they don't. And if they're not good enough for men, then they're certainly not good enough for us. On the other hand, neither is developing a Hotter Shoes catalogue habit.

Here are the rules when it comes to shoes:

- Buy the most expensive you can afford, preferably in the sale, but don't pretend your feet are a tiny bit smaller than they actually are and that the shoes will 'give' a little. They won't. And let's face it, your feet are bigger now than they've ever been (this is due to your arches having collapsed from the weight of carrying you around).

- If in doubt, go to Clarks or any decent department store and find out exactly what size your feet are. Just because you're fifty-three is no reason for a professional not to put that tape measure around your sweaty old pop sock.

- If you like your shoes, look after them: get them re-heeled and re-soled and give them the occasional polish. (Weirdly, polishing your shoes will remind you of your dad and you might have to sit down and have a cry.)

- Finally, never *ever* buy shoes online.

SHOE HINT

A boring old pair of pumps can be given a new lease of life with a fresh pair of laces. You can buy all sorts of colours online – I once jazzed up an old pair of brown suede desert boots with a pair of bright orange laces and at least three people noticed and complimented me, which must be pretty much what it feels like to be Kate Moss.

ODD WARDROBE PIECES THAT WORK

Here are some surprising things that a menopausal woman can get away with:

- Leather biker jackets – but not the Hells Angel's ones covered with loads of badges.
- Blouson bomber jackets – thanks to Mary Berry these have become an acceptable staple in every woman's wardrobe because, regardless of age or size, they work. These are also the kind of things that people with sewing machines can knock up at home, so try and make friends with someone like this and then encourage her to make you lovely things.
- An oversized white shirt – nick the old man's if you don't want to buy your own. Trust me, as long as it's ironed, it'll look great (if it's not ironed, you'll look like a lorry driver coming in from a late-night shift via the pub).
- My other top menopausal fashion tip is to cover everything up with a lovely pinny. Pinnies are great – they can be splattered in gravy, in which case you will look like you know your way around the kitchen, or splattered in paint, in which case you will look arty and bohemian. Either way, they are fantastic disguisers of the gut and, for some reason, men find them a massive turn-on, especially if you've just made them a chocolate cake whilst wearing one.

So remember, girls, when it comes to hot flushes and fabrics, cotton keeps you cool and removable layers make sense. And the most important thing is to make sure you can strip down easily without resorting to ripping seams, tearing at buttons and bursting zips, like some great big hormonal Incredible Hulk.

X-RATED

'Remember sex is cheap and it keeps you warm (mind you, so does making your own soup).' JE

Sex and the menopause is one of those perennials when it comes to newspaper articles about women going through 'the change', and opinions vary according to the journalist and type of publication. Some are all doom and gloom and full of miserable facts about vaginal atrophy with the general advice seeming to be to 'lube up, lie back and hope for the best'; others, written from a more homeopathic point of view, will advise any number of natural remedies to help with dryness from aardvark milk to yam; whilst others still – the more scientific ones – will mention 'vaginal stem cell therapy', which is the latest thing up and down Harley Street and may well be the answer for many women in the future.

Can you imagine what our grandmothers would have made of this? Back then, I think they were told to dab a bit of goose fat down below and keep their fingers crossed. Science marches on though, and now that women are actively seeking help for painful and difficult sex rather than putting up and shutting up, the chances are that real progress will be made.

All these articles and opinions about sex and the menopause have their place, and as different women have different needs it's always reassuring to see your own case history reflected back at you on the page. The more we talk about subjects that were previously thought taboo, the more normal our problems and concerns become.

However, the articles that annoy me the most are those that are written by incredibly glamorous, successful pre-menopausal women – usually in their late forties – who refuse to believe that they will ever feel either undesirable or lacking in libido, insisting that *their* menopause is going to be '*empowering*'.

Well, 'good for you' – and I mean that in the most sarcastic way possible. I really can't stand women who decide what kind of menopause they are going to have before they've even started. Forecasting your menopause is like predicting a baby's birth; in my experience, as soon as you start planning a drug-free water birth, you might as well book yourself in for an emergency Caesarean.

No one has a clue how the menopause is going to affect them, physically, mentally or sexually until they're nether-region deep in it. Ok, so maybe you've got drawers full of the sexiest underwear money can buy, as opposed to the rest of us whose knicker drawer looks like lost property, but nothing can guarantee that you are going to continue to feel as powerful and as sexy as you presume.

There are many reasons why a fifty-year-old woman might feel *empowered*: being the boss, having a great house, pots of money, access to the best gynae care, possessing an electric bike, employing a nutritionist and a personal trainer – in other words, all the stuff us mere mortals don't have. So for these women to insinuate that others who don't feel similarly 'empowered' by the menopause aren't trying hard enough, possibly because they're not exercising right, eating properly or loving themselves enough, is one of my biggest bugbears. (**Warning**: these are the kind of women who get a real kick out of wearing bikinis in their fifties and get slightly competitive with their teenage daughters on the beach. Yuk.)

Possibly, feeling sexy throughout the menopause is easier for those who are blessed with high self-esteem and a great body, but for those of us who are plagued even at the best of times with insecurity and flab issues, the menopause can wreak havoc with how we feel about ourselves sexually. In fact, a great deal of the time the problems we experience sexually are mental as much as physical.

These feelings aren't helped by a media which constantly puts youth on a sexual pedestal whilst knocking those of us over forty on to the old-crone or fat-hag heap. It's very difficult to convince your-self that you're entitled to a sex life when TV, film and advertising continue to insist otherwise.

In the past, it was up to Helen Mirren to singlehandedly fly the flag for the sexy older woman. These days, other older female British celebs whom the press still see as beddable include the gorgeous Kristin Scott Thomas, Nigella Lawson and . . . I'm struggling now, but that's because I've got my *Daily Mail* goggles on! In the real world, of course, there are loads of fifty-plusses who still have it, including quite a few of my mates who continue to be minxes into their sixties, and beyond.

GOING OFF IT

For most of us, sex and the menopause is an incredibly individual and private thing, the real dilemma for many women is that they are no longer sexually compatible with their partners.

Now this is a tricky one and it doesn't matter who is the randy one of the double act and who is the reluctant stooge. The fact is that when one of you is up for it and the other isn't, things can get awkward and embarrassing.

Every night, up and down the country, thousands of men and women pretend to be fast asleep in case the other half should get 'ideas'. Hmmm ... How you get around this predicament is up to you. For a number of women, the problem is a simple case of feeling too physically tired to bother and they find that if they just give it a go (a bit like exercise) it's not that bad and by the time it's all over they've rather enjoyed it, and might even do it again next week!

Some might turn to couples counselling and others might try getting pissed to see if that helps. (It might, but it's not the best solution.)

Weirdly, in 2020 publicly admitting to not enjoying sex is one of the last taboos. We are oh so tolerant of everything else, but we fall down when it comes to acknowledging that, for many people, sex is just not their thing. A bit like golf.

Of course, as with golf, if you don't like it and your partner really does, you do run the risk of him going off and playing with someone else. This is something you have to weigh up. Some couples can survive the extra-marital golf playing, but others can't.

'Why can't they play golf on their own?' I hear you cry. Exactly, but if that is the solution, then you can't complain if you come home and find him practising his swing in the sitting room.

My friends fall into many camps when it comes to sex: some find no longer having to worry about using contraception incredibly liberating and take full advantage of their new-found infertility. But with a few exceptions, most aren't as rampant as they used to be. Although that said, HRT has put the sparkle back into the duvet doldrums for some.

The truth is that, whilst lots of middle-aged women are happily enjoying a healthy sex life, there are millions doing the deed through gritted teeth and faking orgasms as quickly as possible. Because, for them the alternative is unbearable – i.e. actually owning up to the truth of not really enjoying it and having to deal with any possible sulking and recrimination. This isn't fair, but as a mate of mine once said to me, 'I hate having to defrost the freezer but now and again that needs doing too.'

Long-term relationships aren't the sexual kiss of death for every couple, but for many women who have been with the same 'other half' for decades, it can be hard work maintaining their sexy side. (Especially when he's seen you shit your pants in a mini-cab after that time you went swimming in a contaminated lake.) Ditto it's hard to see him as some kind of Love God when he leaves his toenail clippings on the coffee table.

Sadly, everyday life isn't very conducive to romance with arguments over who puts the bins out and '*someone*' forgetting to leave money for the window cleaner leading to huffiness and turned backs in bed.

We're all so tired too. Most of us are so knackered that we fall into bed without cleaning our teeth and the next thing we know we've overslept and it's time to stomp off to work again, and so the pattern repeats.

Women feel hugely guilty about not fancying sex, but the fact is that some of us couldn't care less if we never did it again. The thing about sex is that it's a bit like making your own pastry: you know you should, but you're just not sure if you can be bothered.

This can be difficult to understand for those for whom sex still plays a big part in their lives. After all, the kids have left home, you can do what you like, where you like, when you like. It's just that you might prefer to do some gardening or finish that book or wash your hair!

Of course, there are millions of men who struggle too and for them the obvious physical side effects of ageing are tricky to cope with. Impotence (which basically means the inability for a man to achieve either an erection or an orgasm) is an impossible problem to hide, which is why some chaps get so uptight about it. Again, science stepped in some years ago with the introduction of Viagra, which might be good news for some men and women, but not for others. (For me, it's the ads for Viagra that I find a bit off-putting – the last thing I'd want is the old man making love 'like a teenager again', imagine that? All that fumbling about, missing the target area and worrying about his mum bursting in, no thanks!)

That said, if maintaining a good sex life is important to you, then you might have to be prepared to put the prep in. As my friend Podcast Judith says, 'I just need a lot more notice now'.

RE-IGNITING YOUR SEX LIFE

There are all sorts of things you can do to jump-start your sex life:

- I'm not a big fan of the romantic candlelit bedroom. It's very hard to relax and enjoy yourself when at the back of your mind all you can think about is those curtains going up in flames and having to run out into the street with no clothes on. Subdued lighting, however, is vital – so make sure your bedroom comes with sexy dimmer switches, failing that throw your knickers over your bedside light and with any luck it will cast a nice big shadow over the proceedings.

- Don't go mad and start experimenting with all sorts of different positions, not without warming up first! What we really need is an NHS-approved alternative to the *Kama Sutra* with illustrations featuring all sorts of easy-access angles that won't make your calves cramp or hurt your knees.

- Remember at your age, your blood-sugar levels can suddenly drop, so pop a barley sugar under the pillow for some half-time sustenance should you need it.

- Try and keep the conversation suitably sexy. For example, it's very bad form to interrupt the flow by suddenly asking, 'Did you remember to put the anti-freeze in the car?'

Having said all the above, we all know sex isn't the only way of maintaining intimacy within a relationship. Intimacy can be as simple as a hand squeeze over the breakfast table, an arm around your shoulder in the cinema or a wink across a crowded room. All couples have their own way of showing each other they care, and whilst for some this includes a regular healthy bonk, for others it's picking their partner up from the airport at 4am without whining.

Fortunately, I reckon the vast majority of couples reach some tacit, silent agreement that sex is something that is inevitably going to happen less frequently but that it's nothing to get your knickers in a twist over. And in any case, it's quality and not quantity that really counts.

STIs: RUBBER JOHNNIES AT THE READY

Obviously, not every menopausal woman is in a relationship, long-term or otherwise, and for those who aren't, sex can be something they really miss. Because for every online dating ad that's searching for 'companionship and Scrabble playing', there are probably as many who just want 'a decent shag'. And whilst very few dating biogs are as blunt as this, when 'A physically active fifty-something female seeks a physically active male/female for fun and frolics', I don't think we're talking fell walking.

So at this point, I just need to be very sensible and remind everyone that even though your days of risking an unwanted pregnancy are over (whoop), there is still the possibility of catching a sexually transmitted disease.

It might surprise some people to know that STI diagnoses in the UK's fifty- to seventy-year-old age bracket have risen by more than a third over the last decade. This is thought to be down to rising divorce rates amongst us baby boomers and not bothering with condoms – because . . . well, what's the point? And the point is that many of us are taking our very liberal 1970s attitudes towards sex into our middle years and clocking up multiple later-life partners. Every time we sleep with someone new, we are also sleeping with everyone they have ever slept with (and by 'sleeping with', I mean fucking).

The most common infections for the demographic known as 'the silver singles' are genital warts, chlamydia, herpes and gonorrhoea, with HIV also on the rise.

Although STI infection amongst our age group is still relatively low compared to the youngsters, it's worth getting yourself checked out at your local GUM clinic before embarking on a new relationship. It's a matter of politeness – and if he/she/they aren't prepared to do the same for you, then insist on protection at all times.

PS And never skip a smear test, ladies. Age is no prevention against the HPV virus, which is one of the leading causes of cervical cell changes. Detected early, this can be dealt with before any cancer has a chance to develop.

Basically, have fun, but look after yourselves. Love, Mum x

FINALLY – DIY

We all know you don't need a partner to have a sex life; there's no age limit for wanking (or 'masturbation', as it's more politely known).

When I was about twelve I realized I could bring myself to orgasm by climbing up the bannister rail in my house. I continued this practice for many years, often achieving more pleasure from this mahogany rail than from the boyfriends I was seeing at the time. I also realized a similar thrill could be achieved by climbing up the rope in gym, which soon proved to be the only activity I enjoyed in PE.

Sadly, I think my rope and bannister-rail days are now over – I'm not sure I've got the upper body strength for it any more – but there are alternatives. A quick browse online will take you to special sites dealing in sex aids for older people. And if this doesn't give you a tingle, then you can always have a gander through the Lakeland catalogue to see if there are any handy kitchen implements that could double up as pleasure aids – the banana guard, anyone? Bright yellow, so it's easy to find in the dark and fully dishwasher proof too!

Older and Wider

Seriously, there is nothing wrong with a bit of self-love, though as an audience member once told me during a show, the only drawback to providing your own sexual pleasure is 'when the arthritis kicks in before you've finished'.

YOUTH (AND THE FOUNTAIN OF . . .)

'Sisters, if you want to look younger, then stand next to some-thing older. Hadrian's Wall is ideal.' **JE**

Youth is weirdly fleeting and we never really appreciate it whilst we've got it, but as soon as it's gone we spend the rest of our lives trying to recapture it.

Young people have no idea how beautiful they are. Millions of teenagers and twenty-somethings wake up every day, hating their thighs, worrying about their boobs and wishing they had better skin/hair/teeth. Meanwhile, *we* pass them on the street and think, Look at you, you gorgeous thing.

TURNING BACK THE TIDE

Fiction: You can regain your youthful bloom by drinking many gallons of water a day (so say all those women's magazines).

Fact: Once you've lost your youthful bloom, it doesn't matter how much water you drink, you're never going to get it back. Plus, at your age, you'll spend all your time trying to find the nearest loo.

Older and Wider

I'm sorry to say this, but there is something that happens to a menopausal woman's skin. It loses some of its elasticity and everything begins to sag – tits, chin, jowls. You can help the tits by having your bust measured properly and buying a bra that actually fits and manages to hoik the old girls up a bit. But dealing with the face can be trickier.

For me, the difference between forty-seven and fifty-seven was very cruelly exposed when I tried to get through a machine-operated passport control at Heathrow Airport a couple of years ago with a photo that was over nine years old. Try as I might – and I did . . . about ten times – I could not get the machine to match my passport photo with the actual face the automated lens was viewing. Eventually, due to a bad-tempered queue that was forming behind me, I was hauled over to a security desk where a female passport officer proceeded to tell me, 'It's your face, love; it's not the same as it used to be. That passport photo is really old, see. Happens to us all, love. You get a bit puffy around the eyes, bit chubby around the chops. Add a few wrinkles, a couple of extra chins and the machine say no, haha.' I wouldn't really have minded, but I'd just returned from a week's holiday – I was meant to be looking better.

Dealing with the very visible signs of ageing in the mirror can be difficult, particularly if you've been cute in your time and weren't expecting to turn into a big lady-toad features. The question here is, do you accept the ravages of time or do you try and peel back the years, literally, by having a load of work done? And how much younger can you really look?

From the 'work' I've seen done around London over the past few years, most surgery doesn't make you look younger – it just makes you look weird. I saw a really well-loved TV presenter the other day and for a few minutes I wasn't sure if it was her or her frozen-faced twin. Cross my heart, so far I've resisted the temptation to have any work done whatsoever. Oh . . . you didn't think I had!

On the *Older and Wider* podcast that I do with Judith Holder, quite a lot of our 'women-of-a-certain-age' guests have admitted, both off and on air, to having had a teeny bit of Botox and just a tad of filler. From what I can see, those who have a tiny bit done now and again look the best, and I suspect they all go to the same place, although so far no one has divulged this clinic's number!

Still, I am very ambivalent about having 'tweaks' done. I don't think it makes you look younger, however, as I've said, I do think occasionally it makes you look better. For example, I have a couple of friends who have had hereditary eye bags removed as both were in show business and they were looking really bad in on-screen close-ups. Neither of them looked dramatically different post-surgery – they just looked like they'd had a decent night's sleep.

As a predominantly stage performer, I've always felt that it's vital that my face should be mobile. I'm quite clowny in that respect and in the past, I have always used a great deal of make-up whenever I am gigging to accentuate my features. Since my dry-eye diagnosis, however, I am no longer allowed to wear eye make-up and this depresses me hugely. I try to make up for it by doing a very dramatic lip, and I'm also toying with the idea of at least having my eyebrows tinted, although whether this would be the first step on the slippery slope to getting the whole shebang pinned up and tied around the back of my ears I have no idea.

I think what happens is our faces are a bit like our kitchens, and after years of looking ok (if a bit ordinary) the kitchen suddenly starts looking really tired around the edges. So you either try and spruce it up with a potted plant, maybe a couple of funky pictures (the interior design equivalent of a pair of statement earrings) or you get the experts to come in with a load of scaffolding and give it a complete makeover.

At the moment this is how I feel about my face. I did a telly job recently which involved sitting on the same sofa as Holly Willoughby and catching sight of myself on the monitor. I was suddenly really upset about my jowls and neck – I seem to have lost all definition around my jawline and, as a result, my neck and my face have morphed into one big shapeless lump. To be honest, I don't know whether I need a surgeon or a quantity surveyor.

Of course, losing a couple of stone *would* probably redefine my jawline, but it's very tempting to go for a quick-fix solution rather than starving myself for six months. In reality though, I probably won't do anything because I'm far too mean – and anyway, at the moment it's a toss-up as to which is looking the most knackered: my face or my actual kitchen. So for the time being, I'll stick with a line from my stand-up set: 'I'm not having Botox. The way I see it, if I wanted snake poison running around my system, I'd suck off Boris Johnson.'

All of us struggle to come to terms with ageing, especially when it seems that the last flower of youth fades with the menopause. No wonder women panic; at least men can grow a beard over their non-existent jawline (not that we can't, it's just not socially acceptable).

In fact, growing old as a woman is not really socially acceptable full stop. Youth is where it's at, so no wonder women are bankrupting themselves buying anti-ageing lotions, potions and serums, all promising an elixir of science and magic. According to the side of one bottle of age-defying night cream in the chemist, the mixture boasted a hydrolipidic and biometric double formula, containing twenty different plant oils and turmeric? The cosmetics industry can feed us any old rubbish, and as long as it 'fights the visible signs of ageing' and promises to help eradicate 'fine lines and wrinkles' we'll lap it up. Animal placenta in your moisturizer, girls? Pop it in a tiny pot, put a big cardboard box around it and it will retail for a couple of hundred quid.

Back in 2018, I wrote a furious column for the *Independent* on this very subject:

I'm so tired of all this guff aimed at the fifty-plus female market. It's like they expect us to behave like a load of lobotomized sheep and flock to the beauty counters to part with our hard-earned cash so that, God forbid, we don't actually go out on to the streets looking our age. Oh, the shame.

I mean, how dare we actually face the world with our crow's feet and eye bags, not to mention our ghastly turkey-wattle throats?

Tell you what, maybe there should be a curfew so that old women aren't seen in public during the hours of daylight? Maybe we should scuttle like cockroaches in the twilight hours; maybe they should black out the supermarkets so that no one has to see us in the actual flesh; maybe we should wear bells around our disgusting necks?

It's the implicit barrage of criticism I could do without, that constant whispered reminder that comes from all sides: you're old, you're fat, you're ugly. Well, so what?

There are possibly hundreds of thousands of women who are young and pretty and rather boring, but the media doesn't exactly go round screaming this fact into their faces.

For some reason society isn't yelling, 'Why don't you put your eyebrow pencil down and go and learn something useful? Ok, so you've got a thigh gap, what exactly are you going to do with it?'

Dullness and stupidity aren't picked up on as things to be ashamed of and yet getting older is.

I really don't get this, because the thing that terrifies me most about living right here, right now, isn't my face in the mirror, it's the fact this country sets so little store by having any intelligence, knowledge or experience. Hobbies are sneered at, amateur enthusiasms are patronized, but a daft girl who is proud not to read books and hasn't done much beyond fill her phone with selfies is feted for looking fantastic in a bikini.

I'm not pretending that I'm not vain. I hold my tummy in for photos, for heaven's sake, I bleach my hair, and when I was told, after being diagnosed with dry-eye disease, that wearing eye make-up ever again would be very silly, I was devastated, and have compensated ever since with lashings of blusher and lipstick to the point where I probably look a bit mad.

I also use skin cream, religiously, morning and night – without it my face would turn to bark – but I expect it to keep my skin supple, not perform some magic clock-turning-back trick.

Skin is skin and your own skin depends on many factors, mostly genetic, some lifestyle choices (we all know heavy drinking and smoking take their toll, as do worry and not sleeping).

Anyway, it's not just your face that gives your age away, there's loads of other stuff: clicky knees, pterodactyl hands, that grunting noise you make when you get out of a chair and, possibly the biggest give away of all, no longer being able to giggle in a girlish way, without sounding insane.

Neither are the tell-tale signs of ageing all physical. There are other more subtle giveaways including your favourite Bunty characters, the Blue Peter presenters (and dog) you grew up with and the faces of the pop stars on your teenage bedroom wall. It's the food you ate when you came home starving from school and what your guides uniform looked like, it's the colour of your first nail varnish (Miners 'murky mauve') and the first record you ever bought (Freda Payne's 'Band of Gold'). It's how old you were when you first saw David Bowie on *Top of the Pops* and the car your dad gave you lifts in. It's in your conversation, in the hopes and fears for your parents and kids, it's about how much time you've got left on your mortgage and how long you've been listening to *The Archers*.

Your age is ingrained. It certainly isn't skin deep. And it's about time the cosmetics industry accepted that, laid off trying to make us all feel so crap and stopped guilt tripping us into buying their phoney science.

And there you have it, ladies: how I feel about the anti-ageing industry bollocks in a nutshell (or rather, quite a long rant).

And for those who say age is just a number and whine on about being as young as they feel – grow up, act your age, own it. Let the youth have their fashion and festivals and, for God's sake, just don't try and copy them. There are some things that only the truly young can get away with – and they include the following:

- Really sexy dancing – including anything in a club that involves a pole (just because you can doesn't mean you should)
- Glittery phone cases (unless you're being really ironic, of course)

- Fairy wings and face paint (even if having your face painted like a tiger does take years off you, stop it)
- Hair bobbles and high bunches (not cute, it's tragic)
- Hats with ears on them (as above)
- Micro scooters (exceptions will be made for grandmothers who have dropped grandchildren off at school and are lumbered with taking the bloody thing home)
- Taking helium/any recreational drugs (you never know what's going to mix badly with your statins); obviously, you may have cannabis for medicinal purposes
- Watching cool youth stuff on Netflix and talking about it in public (cringe)
- Wearing toe/belly-button rings (sorry – these will be confiscated)
- And finally, using street slang – 'shut it, Grandma'!

So youth is great. Your tits and arse defy gravity and your neck hasn't got those tortoise-like wrinkles. But remember the flipside – remember how nuts you felt most of the time, how you had no idea what you were going to do or how you were going to make a living or where you were going to live? There's still a load of stuff that freaks me out about life post-sixty, but I wouldn't turn the clock back for the world.

z

ZZZZZZZZZzzzzzzzzzzzzzzzzzzzz

'*The menopause has turned me into a giant toddler: I need regular naps, otherwise I get overtired and start biting people.*' **JE**

The menopause is tiring, physically and mentally and this can be for many reasons:

1. Because you didn't get any kip last night. You were too hot and sweaty – and the night before and the night before that. In fact, you haven't really slept since last August bank-holiday Monday.
2. Being in a foul temper. God, anger is exhausting, especially if your temper manifests itself in clenching your jaw. Jaw clenching is really tiring; believe me, I know – as does my friend Podcast Judith who during one particularly aggressive phase of the menopause was prescribed a mouth guard to prevent her from grinding her teeth during the night!
3. Having to stand up on public transport to get to work because obviously it's more important for a fourteen-year-old boy to have a seat than you and of course you can't make a fuss because you're not *that* old, but even so, you could cry, or spit

or both. Instead you just mumble, 'You rude, selfish little shit' until it's time to get off the bus.

4. Working in a stuffy office and having to get up every two minutes to open the window or turn on the air con because you are having hot flush after hot flush and that silly bint three desks down keeps closing it because she weighs seven stone and starts shivering with cold if the office isn't hotter than an orchid house.

5. Having to listen to people talk shit all day = really tiring.

6. Spending your lunch hour trying on jeans. There is nothing more tiring or depressing than trying on jeans.

7. Because you spent your lunch hour trying on jeans, you missed lunch, and by 2.30 you feel faint with exhaustion and hunger and think you might die.

8. You ate the leftover stale birthday cake that's been sitting on the windowsill for three days. It was Donna's thirtieth birthday cake, was in the shape of a unicorn and had a great deal of glitter icing. You shoved it in your gob and an hour later had the worst sugar slump ever.

9. You go to the toilet hoping to die, have a wee and can barely summon the strength to pull up your jeggings.

10. Before you can get home and either rest or die you have to think about what to buy for supper. For the rest of the afternoon all you can think about is whether you've got sausages in the fridge at home, but you can't remember because you have menopausal brain fog. Also you are sick of being the one who decides what to eat every day and you're sick of being the one that cooks it and just the prospect of having to take the bus home, go to the supermarket and cook dinner, makes

you feel so tired that all you want to do is curl up under your desk like a big cat and kip down in the office for the night but apparently, according to Janice in HR, that's against office rules. Fuck Janice.

11. On the bus home you have to stand up all the way again, because the same fourteen-year-old boy is sitting in the same seat playing with his stupid phone, 'selfish bastard'.

12. You stop off for sausages and pick the queue with the pensioner paying in coupons, this takes forty-five minutes and by now your feet have swollen up so much you might have to be cut out of your shoes.

13. When you get home, you find you already have sausages, but they've gone off, so you cook the new ones, but by this point you are so tired you can barely stand.

14. Your teenage children tell you they are vegans as of like now, like today.

15. You throw sausages at the wall and slightly sprain your arm; bedtime can't come soon enough – all you want is sleep, precious, glorious sleep.

16. You fall asleep during *Inspector Morse*. It is the best sleep ever, but your horrible partner wakes you up and says you can't sleep fully dressed on the sofa. You haul yourself up the stairs, leave your clothes in a heap on the floor and crawl into bed. It's only 10pm, and with any luck you could have nine hours solid hours in the sleep bank by morning. You shut your eyes and wait to slip under that soft black velvet blanket of sleep and guess what? You can't. You can't get to sleep – it's worse than trying to orgasm. Whyyyyy, why can't you sleeeeep?

WHY CAN'T YOU SLEEP?

1. Because you are trying too hard and worrying about not sleeping is making you really tense.

2. Because you wake up three times a night needing a wee and it takes you for ever to get back to sleep because your partner is a man and therefore he snores. Remember, it is a medically proven fact that men snore; women simply breathe lightly through the nostrils in order to stay alive through the night – we do not snore.

3. Worry. Night-time is when the fear kicks in big time. You just lie there, trying to put your worries into alphabetical order and then grade them a worry score between one and ten. So far you have twenty-seven worries, with 'squirrels in the attic' meriting the maximum worry score of ten. This is because you just know they're chewing through your electrics and that one day soon the whole place is going to fuse and there will probably be a massive house fire, therefore, it is your job to lie awake in order to keep everyone safe.

4. Because your vagina itches and all you can think about is – your itchy vagina.

5. Because your sheets and pillowcases feel limp and grubby and you know they need washing and ironing but every day you wake up too tired to even think about stripping the bed. It's been over a month now, but don't tell anyone.

WHAT MIGHT HELP?

- Blackout blinds, like during the war.
- New pillows that aren't deeply dribble stained.
- Lavender pillow mist – oh listen, you've heard all this stuff a million times before, but you never know it might work (but then so might a great big glass of red wine).
- A silent partner who doesn't move all night long and breathes really quietly (good luck with that, girls).
- Sex. Worth a try.

But it's not just the physical lack of sleep that makes us tired. We are tired because being menopausal usually coincides with being middle-aged and by the time we're in our fifties, everything is getting old and worn out – your sofa, the curtains in the dining room, your hips and your knees. It seems to take such an effort just to keep things ticking over. And the menopause puts you on an emotional short fuse, so it doesn't take much for you to explode: you lose your bus pass, the dishwasher starts pebble-dashing your crockery, the washing machine begins making a terrible noise, you've got that spinning ball thing on your computer screen, someone has upended a full box of Rice Krispies in the kitchen cupboard and been really lazy about clearing them up, you find a perfectly good packet of ham at the back of the fridge which is now five days beyond its sell-by date, your good white bra accidentally went in a dark wash – and on it goes, day in day out, thousands of tiny little things that once upon a time you'd be able to laugh off, but not any more. Now you just want to sit on the floor and cry.

And because you are tired, you are tired of being taken for granted and underestimated and overlooked and underpaid, tired of skivvying and mopping up after everyone else, tired of being worried about money, your kids, your ageing parents and the fact that even if you had the room, you couldn't deal with your mum and dad moving in anyway. And then there's all the big stuff on top of the mortgage mountain – there's climate change and bees and food waste and single-use plastics and sometimes the world is so overwhelming and everything is so frightening that it's no wonder you occasionally need to take yourself away from the eye of the storm and have a little nap.

NAPS

If you can, nap whenever you need to. Don't feel guilty for having forty winks on the sofa; the world isn't going to come to a grinding halt just because you nodded off for a few minutes. To be honest, I don't need a lousy night's sleep to give me an excuse to nap the next day. I'm a big napper regardless of whether I had my full eight hours or not and when I say nap, I mean I quite regularly conk out for a good hour in the afternoon. Because, let's face it, there's got to be some perks to being a freelance writer and performer and one of them is working from home during the day and never being more than thirty feet away from my bed.

If you struggle to switch off sufficiently to power nap, then in my experience, it's easiest to nod off when you shouldn't. Hence some of my best catch-up kips have been in the cinema and the theatre. This might be a slightly pricey last resort, but if you are really desperate for a couple of hours' solid sleep, then book yourself a ticket to see something that you have absolutely no interest in and prepare to nod off within ten minutes – bad Shakespeare productions or sci-fi movies are my go-to cultural Mogadon.

PS Try not to snore really loudly during the quiet bits and, whatever you do, do not attempt this trick during one of my shows.

TAKING A BACK SEAT

Ok, so we're tired because not only are we menopausal but we do too much. So let's cut back, let's 'let go', because doing everything is mostly our fault: we have control issues, we genuinely believe that only we can do everything properly, so we refuse to let anyone else have a go. Of course, the problem with doing everything is that everyone gets used to us doing everything and they forget to even offer to help. Eventually, this makes us angry and resentful, so we have to step back. We have to stop filling lunch boxes for teenagers who are perfectly capable of making their own lunch. The trouble with this is that said teenager will use that massive chunk of leftover beef we were going to mince for a cottage pie just to fill a single sandwich and so the cycle begins again – we take over, we get resentful, we're knackered . . . Well, stop it! it's not easy allowing other people to take charge but in the end it's good for all of us. We can't be in charge of everything for ever. Sometimes we have to come to the conclusion that the world will keep on spinning even if we haven't got our shoulder to it. It can't always be our turn, not all the time. Now and then it's good to let someone else have a go and if they do make a pig's ear of it, imagine how secretly delighted you will be!

OF COURSE, WHAT WE ALL REALLY NEED
IS A HOLIDAY

Trouble is, holidays are spendy and there's always a bit of you wondering if the other hotel would have had a better pool and anyway, you don't want to swim because then you'd have to take your sarong off and why are you still so fat when you've been to zumba three times . . .

Ok, so what I'm suggesting instead is that you occasionally take yourself on a virtual holiday. You don't need to actually go anywhere – you can stay at home – but instead of doing all the stuff you don't want to do, you only do the stuff you do want to do, whether that's taking yourself off for a ten-mile hike in the rain, closing the curtains and watching Gene Kelly movies or having your trotters done by the woman in the market who takes a cheese grater to your heels. You don't have to spend a fortune to be nice to yourself; you just need to remember to do it now and then.

It's important to let yourself off the hook sometimes, ladies because one thing is for sure, being menopausal 'ain't for cissies'. Which is why men are designed not to go through it – poor things just couldn't cope!

AND ON IT GOES . . .

Remember, girls, the menopause is not a full stop, it's a punctuation mark. Life goes on. Even though it's a defining moment in your life – a kind of dividing line between being young and, well, being older – let's not forget that the years post menopause can be really brilliant. That's what I'm banking on, anyway. The really tricky stuff is over, the confusion and messiness of getting used to the changes in your body and head have been dealt with and, with any luck, you're metaphorically swimming into calmer waters.

There are also loads of perks to look forward to. For example, when you hit sixty, there are free eye tests and prescriptions, cheaper public transport, gym memberships and even cinema tickets (my local offers free tea, coffee and biscuits to the over sixties, whoop).

Late middle age is potentially where we can really come into our own. Think about all those awesome women who keep on doing what they do and just get better at it: Judi Dench, Helen Mirren, Julie Walters, Sandi Toksvig, Margaret Atwood, Alice Walker, Patti Smith, Oprah Winfrey, Edna O'Brien, Jo Brand, Valerie Amos, Prue Leith. Some of these women are knocking on eighty, but they didn't allow the menopause to stop them in their tracks.

Older and Wider

Older women are the best. We know everything (some of us even know how to use a darning mushroom). And yes, it's occasionally painful to feel sidelined and passed over because, let's be honest here, if we were men, 'late middle age' would be when we were offered all those cushy consultancies and board memberships (think Brian Aldridge in *The Archers*), but there are still plusses. Who cares if we don't go out partying and clubbing like we used to? For starters, home entertainment is so much better than it was ten years ago – what with Netflix and the catch-up channels, plus all those freebie podcasts, there's no earthly reason to be bored of an evening, who wants to be stuck in some dreary Ket hole, when there's all those series of *Brooklyn Nine-Nine* to catch up on.

Life needn't be all antimacassars and jigsaws (though personally, I love a jigsaw). We are ageing differently from previous generations. No one is required to dress from head to foot in beige any more. But on the other hand, neither should we have to deny our menopausal experiences. I find the idea of anyone lying about their age and hormonal status utterly abhorrent – and in any case, your ovaries will always know the truth. It's really important we share our knowledge with the women who are approaching the big M behind us. Because it's only thanks to the women who have broken down menopausal taboos in recent years that we can be open about how we're feeling now.

In the old days, women in the workplace had to battle through the brain fog and hot flushes in silence and with a sense of shame. Not any more. Just as society is getting over the silliness and secrecy that surrounded periods for so long, with men happily slinging tampons for their girlfriends into their grocery baskets, the menopause is beginning to be discussed openly too, be it on the bus, at the hairdresser's or in the office – and we mustn't stop talking about it. The genie can't be allowed back in the bottle.

Every menopausal woman owes it to every other menopausal woman to be honest about how she is feeling and what she is going through, because that's the only way it's going to get easier for women in the future.

As someone who will probably be taking HRT to my grave, I can't in all honesty say that as I hurtle past sixty I'm totally through the menopause. Because there's every chance that if I stop taking the pills and the gel, I will regress back into full menopausal mode (although older friends who have come off the medication say that what they experienced were some very mild symptoms that soon petered out). But the fact is, it's been eight years since I first started feeling like I was losing a grip on the old me. Since then, I can't say that I've emerged like a beautiful butterfly from some hideous old menopausal chrysalis and it would be a lie to say that I've found the 'old me' again. But what I have found is the 'new me' – and you know what? I'm completely cool with that.

Good luck, all.

Much love

Jenny

If you have enjoyed this book, then you might like to try the matching Older and Wider Podcast, which my mate Judith Holder (AKA Podcast Judith) and myself record in a sweat box in Kensal Rise. 'Older and Wider' is available and free to download from iTunes every Friday morning.

Judith and I met when she was producing the Grumpy Old Women TV series, which we then adapted into a succession of touring live shows. This book and the podcast are natural progressions of everything we've shared whilst working together over the past fifteen years, so cheers Judith and long live 'Older and Wider'.

ACKNOWLEDGEMENTS

Big Thanks to Geof and Phoebe for keeping me away from sharp objects when I was at my most unbalanced.

To Jane Sturrock and the Quercus team for letting me say what I wanted and making sure it all made sense.

To Podcast Judith for being my rock and to all my other friends who know what it's like, especially the performing Grumpy Old Women sisterhood.

I would also like to thank everyone who has kept my career going for so much longer than anyone ever expected. I'm a very lucky woman.